HANDBOOK ON INFLAMMATORY BOWEL DISEASE

(VOLUME 2)

(Peer Reviewed Book)

Handbook on Inflammatory Bowel Disease (Volume 2)

(Peer Reviewed Book)

Dr. Khushboo Gupta, Assistant Professor, Trilok Singh TT College, Lakshmangarh, Sikar, Rajasthan, India

Baijnath Das, Assistant Professor, Teerthanker Mahaveer University College of Paramedical Sciences, Moradabad, Uttar Pradesh

Dr. Sparsha Deep EM, Professor & Head, Department of Pharmacology and Chief Coordinator of Clinical Skills & Simulation Lab at Shridevi Institute of Medical Sciences & Research Hospital (SIMS&RH), Tumakuru, Karnataka.

Dr. Supriya, Senior Dietitian &HOD, Mediversal MultiSupar Speciality Hospital, Patna, Bihar, India

Ms Simran Singh, Assistant Professor (Senior Grade) in the Department of Home Science, IIS deemed to be University, Jaipur, Rajasthan India.

Dr. AK Singhal, Associate Professor, Amrita School of Medicine Faridabad, India

HEMAKSHEE PUBLICATION

Handbook on Inflammatory Bowel Disease (Volume 2)

Edition: 2024
ISBN: 978-81-969920-1-9

Published by Hemakshee Publication
Printed and Distributed by pothi.com

HEMAKSHEE PUBLICATION

Sikar, Rajasthan, India

Email: support@hemaksheepublication.com

Website: www.hemaksheepublication.com

Contents

Preface

This book titled **"Handbook on Inflammatory Bowel Disease (Volume 2)"** is primarily intended to be a collection of peer reviewed and plagiarism free chapters written by research scholars, academicians, scientists, doctors and faculty members of their respective fields. Chapters of this book particularly based on topics such as classification of inflammatory bowel disease, IBD and its pathophysiology and morphology, role of nosodes in the treatment of inflammatory bowel disease ant its dietary management, curative treatment of inflammatory bowel disease by allopathy, the role of immunomodulators in inflammatory bowel disease, surgical treatment for IBD, role of residue in IBD, lactose intolerance and IBD: A comprehensive overview and IBD and mental health.

Volume 1 of this book was already published that seems to be the first-ever Indian published document fully focused on **Inflammatory Bowel Disease** and aims to orient the readers about the multidimensional association and impact of inflammatory bowel disease on physiology, psychology and quality of life of an individual.

Chapters of titled **"Handbook on Inflammatory Bowel Disease (Volume 1)"** were particularly based on topics such as etiology differential diagnosis, prevention and treatment of inflammatory bowel disease (IBD); malnutrition and IBD, role of yoga & meditation in IBD, yoga techniques & quality of life in patients with IBD, role of diet in IBD, use of micro-organisms in prevention & treatment of IBD, role of remission diet in IBD and pediatric IBD compass.

We envisage this book to serve as a professional reference for researchers and practitioners in their relevant scientific field. This book will be very useful for students all over in India and Abroad, academicians, medical doctors, dietitians, nutritionists, health care workers, public health specialists, community science specialists, community development professionals, programmers of national and international agencies as well as libraries of relevant collages and institutions.

This book should be of interest to policy makers, bureaucrats, economists and community scientists and can be a reference material for development industry.

This is the seventeenth book in the series of community upliftment. You can see the details of previous books in the section of list of publications at the end of the book.

With great pleasure, we would like to extend our sincere thanks to all the authors of the chapters for reporting their thoughts and experience related to their research and also for patiently addressing reviewer's comments and diligently adhering hectic deadlines to have the book published in timely manner. Their constant support and cooperation has made our task as editors a pleasure. We believe that this book is an important contribution to the community in addressing research work from numerous domains of Inflammatory Bowel Disease.

It is our sincere hope that many more will join us in this time-critical endeavour and this book will stimulate discussions and generate helpful comments to improve future projects.

Happy reading and feedback awaited.

Dr. Khushboo Gupta
Baijnath Das
Dr. Sparsha Deep EM
Dr. Supriya
Ms Simran Singh
Dr. AK Singhal

Introduction

Dr. Khushboo Gupta

Assistant Professor

Trilok Singh TT College

Lakshmangarh, Sikar (Rajasthan)

Email: drkhushboogupta2017@gmail.com

An aberrant immune response to gut microbiota results in recurrent episodes of gastrointestinal tract inflammation, which are the hallmark of a group of chronic illnesses known as inflammatory bowel disease (IBD). The two forms of idiopathic intestinal disease that make up inflammatory bowel disease are distinguished from one another by the location and extent of their involvement in the bowel wall. (i) The mucosa of the colon is diffusely inflamed in ulcerative colitis. Proctitis, or ulcerative colitis that primarily affects the rectum, can also spread to the sigmoid (proctosigmoiditis), beyond the sigmoid (distal ulcerative colitis), or affect the entire colon, including the cecum (pancolitis). (ii) Transmural ulceration of any part of the gastrointestinal system, most frequently affecting the colon and terminal ileum, is a consequence of Crohn's disease. Both conditions are categorised according to their location and degree (mild, moderate, or severe). The three phenotypes of Crohn's disease are penetrating, stricturing, and inflammatory.

Both Crohn's disease and ulcerative colitis include a wide range of extraintestinal symptoms in addition to the GI tract. While the illnesses can be differentiated from one another in the majority of patients. It is impossible to classify IBD because about 10% of patients have identical traits.

There is a hereditary tendency to both conditions; they are both extremely morbid, and none is treatable. Lastly, there is a higher chance of colorectal cancer with both.

Prevalence

Prevalence of IBD increases day by day due to changing lifestyle, dietary habits and environmental factors. Individuals of all age groups are suffering from IBD in India and worldwide but occurrence of IBD in old age is lower as compared to younger age groups. Geographical variances are seen as southern and urban regions of India may have a relatively higher prevalence compared to northern and rural areas. IBD is considered a global disease and its prevalence has been increasing over the past few decades.

Symptoms (World Gastroenterology Organization)

- Diarrhoea can be linked to mucus or blood; it can also happen at night, and faecal incontinence is a regular occurrence.
- When ulcerative colitis is limited to the rectum, some patients may exhibit constipation.
- Severe urgency, tenesmus, and abdominal discomfort are other typical complaints.

- Pain in the right lower quadrant can be a symptom of Crohn's disease, while pain in the left lower quadrant can be a sign of ulcerative colitis.
- With Crohn's disease, nausea and vomiting are more frequent
- Pallor may be observed, depending on the anaemia;
- Common symptoms include tachycardia, anxiety, fever, and dehydration.
- Severe discomfort, fever, stomach distension, chills, and lethargic behaviour are possible symptoms of toxic megacolon. Because it can be fatal if ignored, this surgical emergency should always be taken into consideration.
- Rectal prolapse, anal fistulas, and abscesses are all possible signs of Crohn's disease.
- On a digital rectal exam, occult blood is frequently seen.
- One may only observe growth regression in children.

Diagnosis

Inflammatory Bowel Disease (IBD) poses a diagnostic challenge due to its complex and heterogeneous nature. Clinical evaluation involves a combination of patient history, physical examination, and laboratory tests. Common symptoms include abdominal pain, diarrhea, weight loss, and fatigue. Diagnostic tools such as endoscopy, colonoscopy, and imaging studies like MRI or CT scans help visualize the extent and severity of inflammation. Biopsies aid in confirming the diagnosis

Management

IBD management includes medical management (anti-inflammatory medications, immunomodulators, biologics and JK inhibitors), nutritional therapy (enteral nutrition and dietary modification), surgical interventions (resections, ileostomy and colostomy).

Recent Trends in Inflammatory Bowel Disease (IBD) Management and Treatment

1. Targeted therapies and precision medicine

- **Biosimilars:** Increased availability of biosimilar medications offers cost-effective alternatives to biologics without compromising efficacy.
- **Personalized treatment plans:** Growing emphasis on genetic profiling and biomarker-guided therapy tailors treatment strategies to individual patient characteristics.

2. Advanced biologics and small molecule inhibitors

- **Next-generation biologics:** Novel biologics with different mechanisms of action, such as anti-IL-23 and anti-IL-12 agents, expand the treatment arsenal.
- **JAK inhibitors:** Small molecule Janus kinase inhibitors like upadacitinib and filgotinib

provide additional options, particularly for patients intolerant to or failing biologics.

3. **Top-down treatment approach**

- **Early intervention:** Shifting towards a "top-down" approach involves initiating more potent therapies earlier in the disease course to achieve faster and sustained remission.

4. **Telemedicine and digital health**

- **Remote monitoring:** Telemedicine facilitates regular check-ins, allowing healthcare providers to monitor patient progress and adjust treatment plans without in-person visits.
- **Mobile applications:** Apps for symptom tracking, medication adherence, and dietary management enhance patient engagement and self-management.

5. **Microbiome-targeted therapies**

- **Fecal microbiota transplantation (FMT):** Ongoing research explores FMT's potential in restoring a balanced gut microbiome, influencing disease activity in IBD.
- **Prebiotics and probiotics:** Proactive use of prebiotics and specific probiotic strains aims to modulate the gut microbiota and improve symptoms.

6. **Patient-centric care**

- **Shared decision making:** Encouraging active involvement of patients in treatment decisions fosters a collaborative and personalized approach.

- **Patient education:** Increased emphasis on educating patients about their condition, treatment options, and lifestyle modifications enhances overall disease management.

7. Surgical innovations

- **Minimally invasive surgery:** Advancements in laparoscopic and robotic techniques reduce postoperative complications and recovery times.
- **Strictureplasty:** For Crohn's disease, innovative surgical approaches like strictureplasty aim to preserve bowel length and function.

8. Nutritional approaches

- **Exclusive enteral nutrition (EEN) optimization:** Fine-tuning EEN protocols and exploring its combination with other dietary interventions for improved efficacy.
- **Enteral nutrition in crohn's disease:** Ongoing research on the role of enteral nutrition in inducing and maintaining remission, especially in pediatric cases.

9. Real-world evidence and comparative effectiveness research

- **Long-term outcomes:** A growing focus on real-world evidence helps evaluate the long-term effectiveness and safety of various treatment strategies beyond clinical trials.

- **Comparative studies:** Comparative effectiveness research guides clinicians in choosing the most appropriate therapy based on real-world outcomes.

Prognosis

The severity of the illness and the responsiveness to treatment determine the prognosis for both UC and CD. The stool markers calprotectin and lactoferrin can be used to identify CD recurrence following surgery. There is evidence to suggest that they can be utilised to forecast flares in the future. However, compared to the general population, people with IBD typically have substantially higher mortality rates. Primary diseases, infections, and respiratory ailments are among the causes of death. Heart illness does not increase the chance of dying from IBD. Lastly, IBD patients have very high psychological morbidity and low quality of life.

For long-term UC patients, screening for dysplasia must continue. For people who have had colorectal cancer for 30 years or longer, the cumulative risk is thought to be as high as 30%. Liver failure is the result of primary sclerosing cholangitis' extraintestinal manifestation.

Impact of IBD on Different body organs

Inflammatory Bowel Disease (IBD), comprising Crohn's disease and ulcerative colitis, primarily affects the gastrointestinal tract (hemorrhage, strictures, colon perforation, anal fistulas, pelvic or perirectal abscesses, toxic megacolon, cholangiocarcinoma, colon cancer).

However, its impact can extend beyond the intestines (extra intestinal, i.e., osteoporosis, deep vein thrombosis, anemia, gallstones, primary sclerosing cholangitis, aphthous ulcers, arthritis, iritis, pyoderma gangrenosum), affecting various organs and systems in the body

1. Gastrointestinal tract

- **Crohn's disease:** Can affect any part of the digestive tract, from the mouth to the anus, leading to inflammation, ulcers, and strictures.
- **Ulcerative colitis:** Primarily involves the colon and rectum, causing inflammation and ulceration of the colonic lining.

2. Joints and musculoskeletal system

- IBD patients may experience arthritis, joint pain, and inflammation, known as enteropathic arthritis.
- Conditions like ankylosing spondylitis and sacroiliitis can occur, impacting the spine and pelvic joints.

3. Skin

- Dermatological manifestations are common, including erythema nodosum and pyodermagangrenosum, characterized by painful skin lesions.

4. Eyes

- Uveitis, inflammation of the middle layer of the eye, is a potential complication in IBD.

- Dry eyes and other eye conditions may also occur.

5. Liver

- Primary sclerosing cholangitis (PSC) is associated with IBD, causing inflammation and scarring of the bile ducts in the liver.
- Hepatic steatosis (fatty liver) and autoimmune hepatitis can also be observed.

6. Kidneys

- IBD-related kidney complications include nephrolithiasis (kidney stones) and amyloidosis.
- Glomerulonephritis, affecting the filtering units of the kidneys, is a rare but serious complication.

7. Cardiovascular System

- IBD patients may have an increased risk of cardiovascular diseases, possibly linked to chronic inflammation.
- Vasculitis, inflammation of blood vessels, can occur in some cases.

8. Lungs

- Pulmonary complications include inflammation, pneumonia, and bronchiectasis.
- Conditions like interstitial lung disease may be associated with IBD.

9. Blood

- Anemia is a common complication due to chronic inflammation, nutritional deficiencies, or blood loss.
- Thromboembolic events may occur, increasing the risk of blood clots.

10. Central nervous system

- Neurological complications are rare but can include peripheral neuropathy, seizures, and cerebrovascular events.

11. Psychological impact

- IBD is associated with an increased risk of mental health issues, including anxiety and depression, affecting the overall well-being of individuals.

Conclusions

In the past two decades, advancements in understanding IBD's underlying mechanisms have transformed diagnosis and treatment paradigms. A personalized approach, integrating medical, surgical, and psychosocial strategies, has become pivotal in optimizing patient outcomes. It's crucial for individuals with IBD to receive comprehensive care involving gastroenterologists and specialists in related fields to manage and address potential complications in different organs.

Ongoing research and the advent of innovative therapies hold promise for further enhancing the management of IBD. Regular monitoring and a multidisciplinary approach can contribute to better outcomes and improved quality of life for those living with IBD.

Biography
(Dr. Khushboo Gupta)

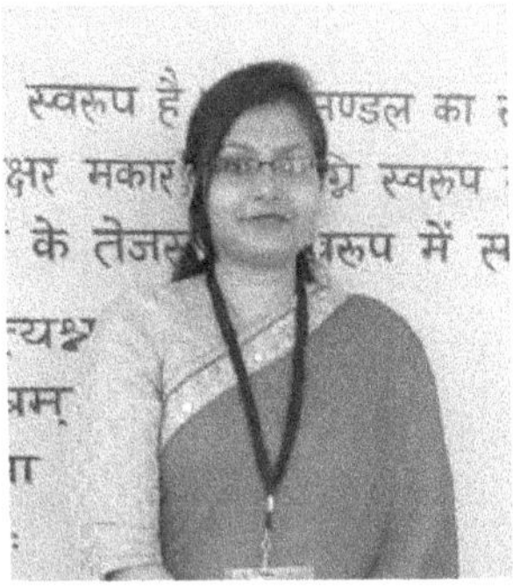

Dr. Khushboo Gupta is a PhD Home Science (Food Science and Nutrition) from Banasthali Vidyapith, Newai, India. She has been teaching subject including food chemistry, food analysis, therapeutic nutrition, human nutrition, human physiology and community nutrition, etc. Presently she is working as Assistant Professor in Trilok Singh TT College, Laxmangarh, Sikar, Rajasthan.

She is MSc Gold medalist and had **cleared UGC-NET and RPSC-SET examination.** Dr Gupta holds Advance Diploma in French Language from Banasthali Vidyapith; Diploma in Naturopathy and Yoga (NDDY) from Gandhi Smarak Prakritik Chikitsa Samiti (Regd.), New Delhi; Certificate in Homeopathic Medicinal System conducted by Vardhman Mahaveer Open University, Kota and Certificate in Statistical Techniques and Applications. She has featured in several programs of All India Radio and Radio Banasthali (FM 90.4).

Dr. Khushboo is actively involved in community activities especially those concerned with self-employment, health and wellness, optimum nutrition and how to improve quality of life of a person and family. She is the keynote speaker and founder of her YouTube channel "Dietitian Ki

Salah" through which she provides education related to optimum health, wellness and nutrition to masses. Dr. Gupta has published about more than 30 research papers in reputed national and international journals; 7 book chapters in different edited books, several news paper and magazine articles related to health, nutrition and new food product formulation. She authored one book related to elderly nutrition; edited **sixteen** books related to community science, food science and nutrition, health and wellness, issues with girls, health for all, sustainable development, food safety and security, breastfeeding and millets for upliftment of the individuals of the society. She presented her research work in more than 26 national and international conferences. Her research is primarily in the area of food processing entrepreneurial skill Inculcation and geriatric nutrition. **The patent office, Government of India has granted a patent to Dr. Khushboo for her research on food formulation using RSM.** Dr. Gupta has successfully completed more than 30 courses on various diverse topics organized by SWAYAM, UNICEF, WHO and Cornell University.

In past she had worked as Assistant Professor (Food and Nutrition) in Modi University, Laxmangarh, Sikar; worked as Master Trainer in Agriculture University, Kota. During her PhD she had worked as UGC- SRF in Banasthali Vidyapith, Newai. One feather in her cap is that she had worked as regular trainee dietitian in dietetics department of Post Graduate Institute of Medical Education and Research (PGIMER), Chandigarh and got her short-term attachment certificate. She won many awards in different seminars and conferences for her contribution in scientific world. Apart from them, she is rewarded with **Teacher Honour award** by Lions Club Kota South (September, 2017); '**Award of**

Honour given by All Rajasthan Qualified Homoeopathic Doctors Association in Homoeopathic Scientific Seminar, 2017, **Excellence Academician Award** given by Akhil Bhartiya Agrawal Mahasabha (Reg), kota Branch (2023) and **Shakti Vandan Award** given by S.R.S.T. College of Education Ova Jahanabad, Bihar in association with Kalindi Prakashan, Ajamgarh, UP.

She is the life member of many reputed institutes i.e. Nutrition Society of India, Indian Dietetic Association, The Indian Science Congress Association and Institute of Scholars and giving her services for upliftment of community.

Biography

(Baijnath Das)

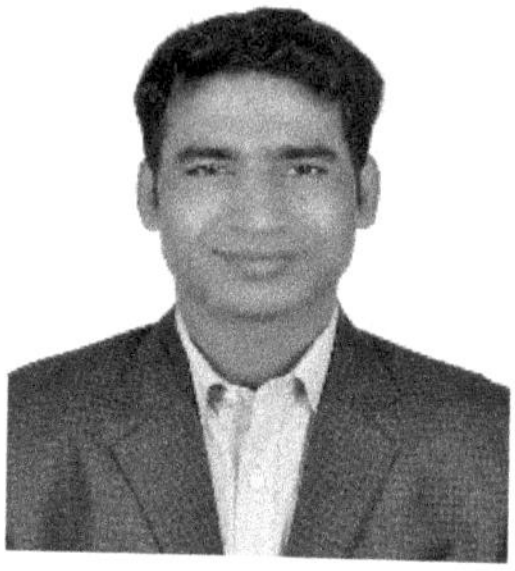

Baijnath Das is a dedicated biochemist with a fervent passion for scientific research and academic exploration. He has continuously pursued academic excellence and made significant contributions to the field of biochemistry. Das earned his Bachelor of Science in Medical Laboratory Technology from Sikkim Manipal University in 2010 and his Master of Science in Medical Biochemistry from the prestigious All India Institute of Medical Sciences (AIIMS), New Delhi, in 2014. Currently, he is pursuing his Ph.D. in Biochemistry at Teerthanker Mahaveer University in India. Das's dedication and academic prowess have been acknowledged through various scholarships and awards. He has published articles in national and international journals, along with various chapters. Additionally, Das has presented posters and attended numerous conferences, showcasing his research acumen. He has also delivered seminars on various topics, demonstrating his depth of knowledge and research skills. Das possesses a diverse skill set in research techniques. His proficiency in these techniques underscores his ability to conduct comprehensive and insightful research. With a rich professional background, Das has served as a Medical Laboratory Technologist at Sunder Lal Jain Charitable Hospital and as a lecturer at various institutes, including Pavitra Institute of Health Science and Swami Vivekananda Subharti University. Currently, he contributes to academia as a lecturer at Teerthanker Mahaveer University, inspiring students and advancing scientific knowledge through his passion for research.

Biography
(Dr Sparsha Deep EM)

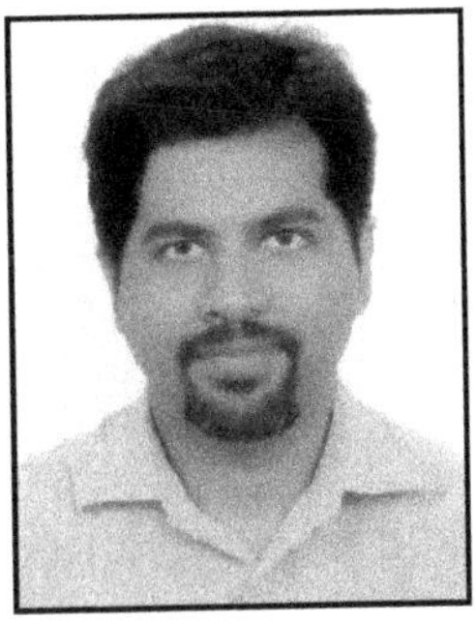

Dr Sparsha Deep EM is currently the Professor & Head, Department of Pharmacology and Chief Coordinator of Clinical Skills & Simulation Lab at Shridevi Institute of Medical Sciences & Research Hospital (SIMS&RH), Tumakuru, Karnataka. He has been serving in the field of medical education, research & clinical practice for the last 15 years. He is a certified Emergency Care & Life Support (ECLS) trainer from Jeeva Raksha Trust, Bengaluru. He has previously given his services in reputed institutions like A J Institute of Medical Sciences & Research Centre (AJIMS&RC), Mangalore, and Govt. Medical College (GMC) Kannur, Kerala.

He has been awarded M-FILIPE (FAIMER) Fellowship from MAHE, Manipal (2021); Advanced Course in Medical Education (ACME) form GMC, Kottayam, Kerala (2016). Dr Sparsha Deep EM has to his credits publications in indexed peer reviewed journals. His areas of expertise are Pharmacotherapeutics; Pharmacovigilance; Clinical Research & ICH- GCP (Good Clinical Practice) and Medical Humanities. He has received Jury Choice award for his presentation on topic 'Clinical simulation in the learning of management of anaphylaxis in medical undergraduates' at JIPMER MEDUCON 2021.

Biography
(Dr. Supriya)

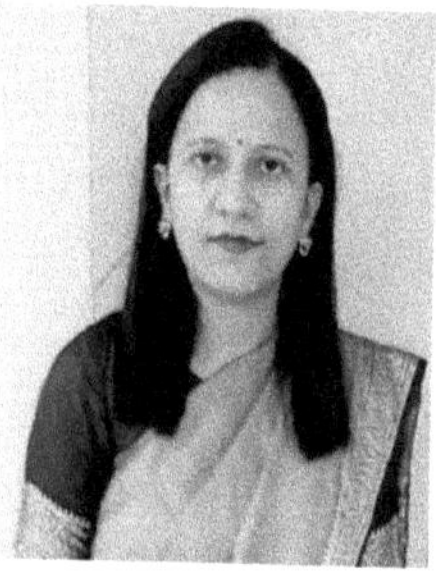

Dr. Supriya, PhD, MSc Food Science & Nutrition (RND, Sadhna Awardee 2024), Senior Dietitian, working as HOD, Dept. of Dietetics & Nutrition, Mediversal Multi Super Speciality Hospital, Patna, CDE, IYCF & Lactation Expert. About 10 years experience in the field of nutrition, research, public health & community nutrition as well. Invited as public health speaker, Keynote speaker, panelist, chairperson and organized various nutrition awareness camp, webinar, etc. Secretary IAPEN India Patna Chapter. Co-Convenor Netprofan Patna Chapter. She clear ESPEN (4 LLL exam in Lyon, France) 2023. She received Dietitian of the year award, ISSN International award. She presented papers in various national and international conferences. Several paper publication in national & International journals. She worked as facilitator/trainer for giving training to FD, staff nurse, medical pg students at CoE, NRC, Patna Medical College & Hospital. Live programme at DD Bihar on the occasion of world breast feeding week, 2019. Organizing committee member in various conference and seminar at Patna. Certified Diabetes Educator (NDEP IYCF Master training. Professional Membership of IDA, NSI, IAPEN, ISPEN, Netprofan, RSSDI.

Biography
(Ms Simran Singh)

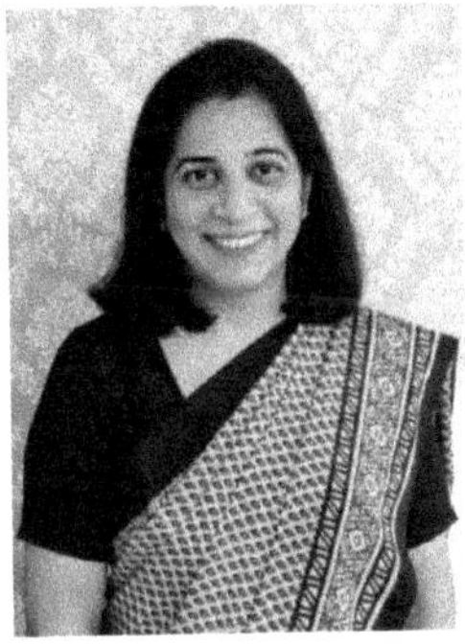

Ms Simran Singh is presently working with IIS deemed to be University, Jaipur as Assistant Professor (Senior Grade) in the Department of Home Science and has been teaching Food Science and Nutrition since 2001. She has also worked at senior positions at Kukreja Institute of Hotel Management and Catering Technology and Institute of Hotel Management Applied Nutrition at Dehradun. Her key research areas are Clinical Nutrition, Food Product Development, Women health, Junk foods, Childhood and Adolescent Obesity and role of Nutrition in Non-Communicable Diseases. Several students have undertaken their post graduate research under her supervision. She has also been trained in Bariatric Nutrition.

She has published in many scientific journals, authored books, served as book editor, written book chapters and contributes articles in magazines and newsletters regularly. Her two patents have got published recently. She has also been on the panel for Developing Mineral Mix for Mid- day Meal scheme in Uttarakhand. Besides, she is also involved in providing consultancy to a nutrition-based start-up in Ahmedabad and development of a health app. She is a life member of Indian Dietetic Association, Home Science Association of India and professional member of Universal Society of Food and Nutrition.

Biography
(Dr. AK Singhal)

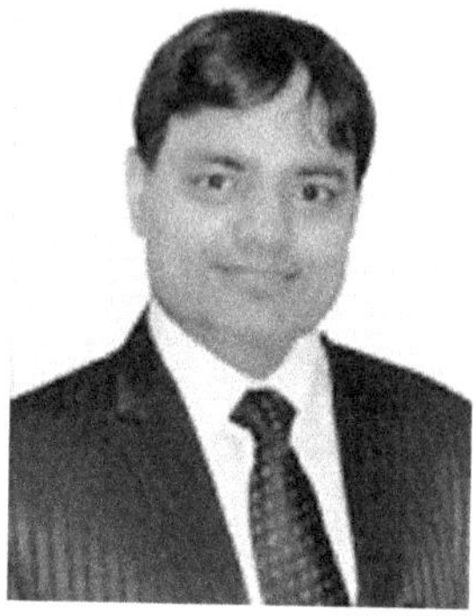

Dr. AK Singhal is a currently working as Associate Professor at Amrita School of Medicine Faridabad. He is distinguished Medical professional renowned for her groundbreaking contributions to both medical education and clinical practice. With a career spanning over decades, Dr. Singhal has left an indelible mark on the field of medicine through his tireless dedication to teaching, innovative research, and compassionate patient care.

List of Contributors

1. **Baijnath Das** Assistant Professor, Teerthanker Mahaveer University College of Paramedical Sciences, Moradabad, Uttar Pradesh.
2. **BR Abha Ayushree** Assistant Professor, PG Department of Home Science, Rama Devi Women's University, Vidya Vihar, Bhubaneswar
3. **Dr Vijaita Gaur,** Principal, SBN College of Education, Shri Madhopur
4. **Dr. (Prof.) Navneet Kumar,** Professor, Teerthanker Mahaveer University College of Paramedical Sciences, Moradabad, Uttar Pradesh.
5. **Dr. Chetna Rochani, MD (Hom),** PG-FHPC, Consulting Homoeopathic Physician, Vadodara, Gujarat, Associate Professor & HOD, Department of Pathology, P P Savani University, Kosamba, Surat.
6. **Dr. Jyotirmayee Udgata,** Associate Professor, PG Department of Home Science, Rama Devi Women's University, Vidya Vihar, Bhubaneswar
7. **Dr. Nishma Singh,** Associate Professor, Shaheed Baba Deep Singh Department of Home Science, Swami Vivekanand Subharti University, Meerut (UP)
8. **Dr. Praveen Katiyar,** Assistant Professor, School of Health Science, CSJM University Kanpur

9. **Dr. Shalu Nehra,** Assistant Professor, Shaheed Baba Deep Singh Department of Home Science, Swami Vivekanand Subharti University, Meerut (UP)

10. **Dr. Vijaykumar Gopaldas Rajani,** BE (Mechanical), D.N.Y.S, Consulting Naturopath, Vadodara, Gujarat

11. **M. Narmadha,** Department of Biotechnology, Prathyusha Engineering College, Tiruvallur 602025, Tamil Nadu

12. **Monalisha Munda,** Assistant Professor, PG Department of Home Science, Rama Devi Women's University, Vidya Vihar, Bhubaneswar

13. **Mori Hetshi Pravinbhai,** Student, P P Savani University, Kosamba, Surat

14. **Ms. Shailendri Kushwaha,** Ph.D. Scholar, School of Health Science, CSJM University Kanpur

15. **Prof. Ruchi Kant,** Professor, Teerthanker Mahaveer University College of Paramedical Sciences, Moradabad, Uttar Pradesh.

16. **Raman Kumar,** Bachelor's Student of B.Sc. MLT, Teerthanker Mahaveer University College of Paramedical Sciences, Moradabad, Uttar Pradesh.

17. **S. Shobana,** Department of Biotechnology, Vel Tech Rangarajan Dr. Sagunthala R&D Institute of Science and Technology, Avadi-600062, Tamil Nadu.

18. **S.G. Nandhika Jothi,** Department of Biotechnology, Prathyusha Engineering College, Tiruvallur 602025, Tamil Nadu

19. **Shivam Agarwal,** Assistant Professor, Teerthanker Mahaveer University College of Paramedical Sciences, Moradabad.

20. **Vaghela Archana Gopalbhai,** Student, P P Savani University, Kosamba, Surat

21. **Vasani Ruta Kiritbhai,** Student, P P Savani University, Kosamba, Surat

If readers have any query related to any chapter of the book, kindly contact with the corresponding author of the chapter. Authors of the chapters are solely responsible for their work.

1.

Classification of Inflammatory Bowel Disease (IBD)

Dr. Jyotirmayee Udgata[1], BR Abha Ayushree[2], Monalisha Munda[2]

Associate Professor[1], Assistant Professor[2,]

PG Department of Home Science, Rama Devi Women's University

Vidya Vihar, Bhubaneswar-751022

Email: udgatajyoti@yahoo.com

Abstract

Inflammatory Bowel Disorders (IBD) are chronic illnesses with relapsing and remitting clinical patterns, such as Crohn's disease (CD) and ulcerative colitis (UC). The phenotypic of IBD varies greatly. There are other immune-mediated illnesses that appear concurrently with IBD but are not yet regarded to be part of the IBD spectrum.However, given on the etiology, pathogenetic pathways, clinical presentation, and disease history, IBD most likely reflects a broad illness spectrum. There are overlaps between IBD and other immune-mediated or chronic inflammatory illnesses. The differential diagnosis, on the other hand, might be problematic. Endoscopy, coupled with histology, is important in disease evaluation. A comprehensive taxonomy of IBD is proposed.

Keywords: Auto-immune disorder, Inflammatory Bowel Disorders, Crohn's Disease, Ulcerative Colitis, Immune-mediated illness

1. Introduction

There are two forms of inflammatory bowel disease (IBD): Ulcerative colitis (UC) and Crohn's disease (CD). CD and UC have unique clinicopathological characteristics.Clinical, imaging, endoscopic, and histologic features are used to identify inflammatory bowel disease (IBD)[1].While broad mucosal inflammation starting in the rectum characterises classic UC, transmural, granulomatous, and skip lesions can be seen in any part of the GI tract in classic CD[2].

The term "inflammatory bowel disease" (IBD) describes a group of inflammatory conditions affecting the colon and small intestine, the most prevalent of which are Ulcerative colitis (UC) and Crohn's disease (CD) [3].Although ulcerative colitis mostly affects the colon and rectum, Crohn's disease usually affects the small and large intestines, as well as the mouth, oesophagus, stomach, and anus[4][5][6].

In the past, Crohn's disease (CD) and ulcerative colitis (UC) were distinguished as two types of inflammatory bowel diseases (IBDs). However, at the 2005 World Congress of Gastroenterology in Montreal, a group of investigators presented a new clinical categorization for both CD and UC. This categorization has significantly changed the landscape of IBD treatment. Despite advancements in our understanding of the disease and the availability of more therapy options, we still face significant limitations in achieving successful treatment outcomes. One of the reasons for this is the heterogeneity of IBD, as there is no consistent phenotype for CD or UC. The current clinical categorization methods are too simplistic and do not capture the full complexity of the disease. Therefore, it is necessary to thoroughly review the existing categorization systems based on a deeper understanding of IBD. In this book chapter, we will shed light on the major clinical variables that contribute to the heterogeneity of IBD, discuss the limitations of current classification algorithms, propose potential improvements, and outline goals for future research in this field.

2. Causes

IBD is a complicated illness caused by the interplay of environmental and genetic variables, which results in immune reactions and gut inflammation.[4]

2.1. Diet

Although those who have IBD are interested in food, little is known about how their diets may affect them. Recent research has demonstrated that IBD patients require dietary counseling. Patients should be urged to follow evidence-based diets that include monitoring for the objective resolution of inflammation.[22][23]

A study conducted in 2022 revealed that diets rich in fruits and vegetables, while being low in processed meats and refined carbohydrates, and high in water consumption for hydration, were found to be linked with a decreased likelihood of experiencing active symptoms of inflammatory bowel disease (IBD). However, it was observed that an increased consumption of fruits and vegetables alone did not lead to a reduction in the risk of symptoms associated with Crohn's disease.[24]

There exists a correlation between dietary habits and an elevated susceptibility to ulcerative colitis. Individuals situated within the uppermost tertile of the wholesome eating regimen, for example, exhibited a noteworthy reduction of 79% in the occurrence of ulcerative colitis.[25]

The prevalence of gluten sensitivity is high among individuals with inflammatory bowel disease (IBD) and has been associated with exacerbations. Specifically, research has revealed that 23.6% of patients with Crohn's disease and 27.3% of patients with ulcerative colitis exhibit gluten sensitivity.[26]

Consuming a diet rich in protein, especially animal protein, and/or a diet high in sugar has the potential to elevate the likelihood of developing inflammatory bowel disease and experiencing relapses.[27][28]

2.2. Bile acids

Recent data indicates that bile acids have a noteworthy involvement in the etiology of inflammatory bowel disease (IBD). In particular, primary bile acids, including cholic acid and chenodeoxycholic acid (as well as their conjugated forms), are found in greater abundance in individuals with IBD. Conversely, secondary bile acids, such as lithocholic acid and deoxycholic acid, are less prevalent in this population.[29]

2.3. Microbiota

Changes in the gut microbiome may contribute to inflammatory gut disorders due to the interaction between microbial symbiosis and immunity.[30] Patients with inflammatory bowel disease (IBD) exhibited a notable decrease in the biodiversity of commensal bacteria, with a reduction of 30-50 percent. This decline was particularly observed in Bacillota, specifically Lachnospiraceae, and Bacteroidota. This finding provides additional evidence supporting the significant role of gut flora in the development of inflammatory bowel disease. Moreover, it was observed that IBD patients were more prone to having received antibiotic treatment within the 2-5 years preceding their diagnosis, further emphasizing the importance of gut microbiota in the causation of this condition.[31] Environmental factors, such as the presence of concentrated milk fats commonly found in processed foods and confectionery, as well as the consumption of oral medications like antibiotics and oral iron preparations, have the potential to alter the composition of enteral microorganisms.[32]

The mucosal microbiota of the large intestine in patients with active inflammation of inflammatory bowel disease (IBD) has been found to be associated with pro-inflammatory changes in the host epigenome. Despite extensive multinational research, no single microbiological biomarker of IBD has been identified, suggesting that the disease is not caused by a single microorganism.

2.4. Breach of intestinal barrier

The impairment of the intestinal epithelium's integrity is a crucial factor in the pathogenesis of inflammatory bowel disease (IBD).[35] The malfunctioning of the innate immune system due to aberrant signaling via immune receptors known as toll-like receptors (TLRs), which triggers an immune response to molecules that are commonly shared by various pathogens, plays a role in the development of acute and chronic inflammatory processes in IBD colitis and related malignancies. [36] Changes in the composition of the intestinal microbiota play a significant role as an environmental factor in the development of Inflammatory Bowel Disease (IBD). Detrimental alterations in the intestinal microbiota trigger an inappropriate and uncontrolled immune response, leading to damage to the intestinal epithelium. These disruptions in the critical barrier of the intestinal epithelium allow for the infiltration of additional microbiota, which subsequently provoke further immune responses. IBD is a complex disease influenced by multiple factors, yet it is partly driven by an exaggerated immune response to gut microbiota, resulting in defects in the function of the epithelial barrier.[37]

2.5. Oxidative stress and DNA damage

Pereira *et al.* conducted a comprehensive review of various studies, which collectively suggest that oxidative stress and DNA damage are likely to play a significant role in the pathophysiology of inflammatory bowel disease (IBD). The researchers observed a notable increase in oxidative DNA damage, as indicated by elevated levels of 8-OHdG, in patients with IBD compared to control subjects.

Furthermore, the levels of oxidative DNA damage were found to be significantly higher in inflamed mucosa compared to non-inflamed mucosa[38]

2.6. Genetics

For more than a century, the existence of a genetic element in the development of inflammatory bowel disease (IBD) has been acknowledged. Furthermore, the genes linked to IBD are more prone to be linked to anxiety, neuroticism, and depression.[39][40].

Research that has contributed to the understanding of genetics includes studies of various ethnic groups such as Ashkenazi Jews and Irish, as well as familial clustering, epidemiological studies, and twin studies. The advent of molecular genetics has significantly expanded our understanding of the genetic basis, particularly in the past decade. In 2001, the first gene linked to IBD was identified as NOD2.

The two primary types of inflammatory bowel disease are Crohn's disease and ulcerative colitis (UC). These diseases are classified as autoimmune diseases, wherein the body's immune system attacks elements of the digestive system.

Other forms of IBD, which are not always classified as typical IBD, are accounted for by accounting for fewer cases. These include microscopic colitis, which is subdivided into collagenous colitis and lymphocytic colitis, diversion colitis, Behçet's disease, early onset IBD, and indeterminate colitis.

Currently, there are no known disease-specific markers in the blood that allow for the reliable differentiation of patients with Crohn's disease and ulcerative colitis. The distinguishing factor between these two conditions lies in the location and characteristics of the inflammatory changes. Crohn's disease can impact any part of the gastrointestinal tract, spanning from the mouth to the anus, with the presence of skip lesions. However, the majority of cases originate in the terminal ileum. On the other hand, ulcerative colitis is confined to the colon and rectum. From a microscopic perspective, ulcerative colitis is limited to the mucosa, which refers to the epithelial lining of the gut. In contrast, Crohn's disease affects the entire thickness of the bowel wall, resulting in transmural lesions. Additionally, Crohn's disease and ulcerative colitis exhibit varying degrees of extra-intestinal manifestations, such as liver issues, arthritis, skin manifestations, and eye problems.

The phrase inflammatory bowel disease refers to three illnesses that share symptoms but differ clinically.

• Chron's disease • Ulcerative colitis• IBS (Irritable Bowel Syndrome).

Mucosal tissue lesions occur in the first two cases, and recurrent removal of the damaged parts of the intestine occurs in the third, all of which result in typical, comparable symptoms.

3. Aetiology

Ulcerative colitis is a condition that produces inflammation and ulcers in the rectum and colon lining. Ulcers arise when inflammation kills the cells that normally lining the colon, causing it to bleed and create pus. Inflammation of the colon also causes it to empty often, resulting in diarrhea. **(Image courtesy of right health)**

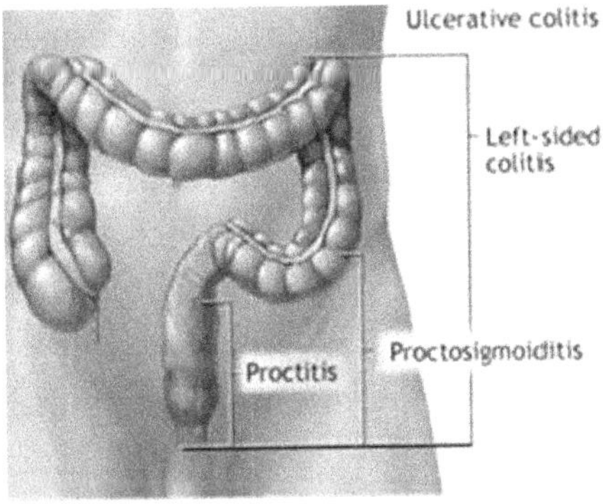

Crohn's disease, also known as regional enteritis, is an inflammatory bowel disease that can affect any section of the gastrointestinal system from the mouth to the anus, resulting in a wide range of symptoms. It typically causes stomach discomfort, diarrhoea (which may be bloody if the inflammation is severe), vomiting, or weight loss, but it can also cause skin rashes, arthritis, eye irritation, weariness, and lack of attention. **(Image courtesy of right health)**

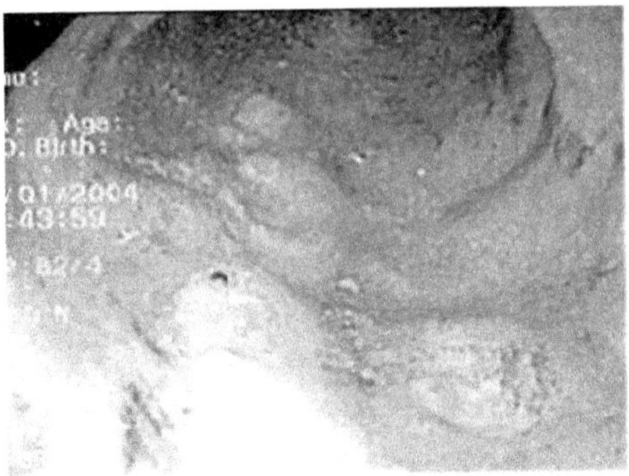

Ulcerative colitis and Chron's disease both have serious nutritional effects. They can be distinguished by two factors.

Chron's disease can arise in any portion of the gastro intestinal system, including the colon, small intestine, and colorectal area. Ulcerative colitis affects just the colon and rectum.

The nature of tissue alterations in Chron's disease is chronic inflammation that can affect any portion of the intestinal wall. This frequently results in the creation of strictures and fistulas. The inflammatory alterations in ulcerative colitis are acute and only remain for a short time. The modifications are also limited to the intestine's mucosal and submucosal tissue layers.

4. Clinical signs and symptoms

Chronic, bloody diarrhea is the most prevalent clinical symptom. Ulceration of the mucous membranes of the intestines causes anorexia, edema, anemia, negative nitrogen balance, electrolyte abnormalities, and other complications. Weight loss is rather frequent.

5. Management

The emphasis in the treatment of these two disorders is on restoring appropriate nutrition. Antibacterial, anti-inflammatory, and corticosteroid drugs are given in addition to supportive treatment. Nutritional supplements should be given to avoid nutrient deficits. Local trauma to inflamed regions must be avoided. Medium chain triglycerides are well tolerated and can be combined with a protein, energy, mineral, and vitamin-rich, low-residue diet.

6. Inflammatory bowel disease

The term "Inflammatory Bowel Disease" is commonly used to describe a persistent inflammatory state of the intestine. This term encompasses three distinct conditions that share similar symptoms but have varying underlying clinical issues. These conditions are: **1. Ulcerative colitis 2. Crohn's disease 3. Short bowel syndrome**

Ulcerative colitis is the designated term for an illness characterized by inflammation in the rectum that extends into the colon, while sparing the right colon and small intestine from damage. However, Crohn's disease presents itself as an inflammatory disorder that impacts either one or multiple extensive portions of the small or large intestine. This leads to inflammation that extends from the mucosa to the serosa.

To elucidate the dissimilarities between ulcerative colitis and Crohn's disease, the following distinctions can be highlighted:

1) The inflammatory process in Crohn's disease affects different parts of the gastrointestinal (GI) tract, such as the small intestine, colon, and even the colorectal area. On the other hand, ulcerative colitis only causes inflammation in the left colon and rectum.

2) In Crohn's disease, the inflammatory process impacts the complete thickness of the small intestinal wall, resulting in the creation of strictures that can lead to blockages or the emergence of fistulas. Conversely, in ulcerative colitis, the inflammatory process is confined to the mucosa and submucosal tissues of the colon and usually endures for a few weeks.

6.1. Etiology

Though hereditary variables, immunological mechanisms, bacterial or viral agents, and sugar (excess) and low fiber consumption have been identified as plausible mechanisms, sugar (excess) and low fiber intake have also been implicated, particularly in Crohn's disease.

The following section summarizes the symptoms and consequences of inflammatory bowel disease.

6.2. Symptoms

Inflammatory bowel diseases are associated with various symptoms, such as abdominal cramping, diarrhea, steatorrhea, obstruction caused by the intake of bulky foods, and malnutrition. What are the factors contributing to malnutrition in these disease conditions? Let's explore.

6.3. Causes of malnutrition in inflammatory bowel disease

There are various factors that can contribute to malnutrition in patients. These factors encompass reduced oral intake, which can be caused by disease-induced symptoms like abdominal pain, diarrhea, nausea, and anorexia. Malabsorption can also occur due to multiple factors, including decreased absorptive surface area, bile salt deficiency, bacterial overgrowth, and the use of specific medications. Furthermore, increased secretion and nutrient losses may transpire as a result of gastrointestinal blood losses, electrolyte imbalances, and trace mineral deficiencies. Patients may also experience heightened nutrient requirements due to inflammation, fever, increased intestinal cell turnover, and haemolysis. Certain medications can impede nutrient absorption, such as corticosteroids, which hinder calcium absorption and protein metabolism, sulfasalazine, which obstructs folate absorption, and cholestyramine, which interferes with fat-soluble vitamin absorption. Patients may also display deficiencies in folate, vitamins A, C, and D, as well as low serum levels of zinc, copper, and iron. Addressing these factors is crucial to prevent malnutrition and promote optimal health in patients.

6.4. Nutritional management of inflammatory bowel disease

The core principles of nutrition management entail guaranteeing sufficient fulfillment of nutritional needs and reducing strain on the inflamed or narrowed section of the intestine.

Individuals admitted to the hospital for Inflammatory Bowel Disease (IBD) are commonly prescribed a "bowel rest" regimen. This regimen entails limiting oral consumption to clear liquids and low residue meals to alleviate symptoms and decrease bowel activity while recovering. The primary goals of this regimen are as follows:

1. To decrease the workload of the bowel and allow it to rest.

2. To minimize mechanical stress caused by the movement of food.

3. To reduce the secretion of diet-related substances (such as acid and enzymes) that may worsen inflammation.

4. In order to ensure an adequate intake of protein and calories, it is essential to provide a diet that is abundant in these nutrients, enabling children and adolescents to maintain or regain weight and promote growth. Furthermore, due to the nutritional deficiencies, impaired absorption, and heightened requirements associated with

this condition, it is imperative to supplement their diet with multivitamin preparations, ideally containing 1-5 times the Recommended Daily Allowance.

It is important to avoid excessive emphasis on fiber intake in individuals with strictures, as this may lead to obstruction. In cases of Crohn's disease, steatorrhea (excessive fat in the stool) is more likely due to ileal resection. This can result in the formation of calcium-fatty acid complexes and increased excretion. It may also lead to losses of magnesium (Mg) and zinc (Zn). Steatorrhea also enhances the absorption of oxalate, which can contribute to higher levels of oxalate in the body. Moreover, this state is distinguished by an elevated attachment of fatty acids to calcium, resulting in a greater availability of oxalate for absorption within the gastrointestinal tract. Fatty acids also enhance the permeability of oxalate through the intestinal mucosa. Therefore, it is recommended to reduce fat intake and supplement with calcium, magnesium, and zinc to address these issues.

In conclusion, a formal approach to nutrition management in patients with IBD involves ensuring nutritional adequacy and minimizing stress on the inflamed or constricted section of the intestine. This is achieved through a "bowel rest" regimen that restricts oral intake, clear liquids, and low residue meals. Additionally, a high protein and calorie diet is recommended, along with supplementation of multivitamins to address nutritional deficiencies. It is important to avoid excessive fiber intake in individuals with strictures, and to address issues such as steatorrhea and increased oxalate absorption

7. Ulcerative Colitis

By reading the following case, you will have a thorough understanding of ulcerative colitis.

Varun, a 48-year-old individual, enjoyed a lengthy and prosperous career within the computer industry. His business endeavors consumed his life, as he dedicated extensive hours and seldom took a break, even on Sundays, when engrossed in significant contracts. Upon successfully completing a transaction, Varun experienced immense joy and celebrated his accomplishments at his preferred Chinese restaurant. However, due to his demanding work schedule, he often resorted to ordering his beloved Chinese cuisine, which unfortunately resulted in frequent episodes of diarrhea. Regrettably, his most recent encounter with this ailment was particularly distressing. For two consecutive nights, Varun suffered from illness, enduring painful cramps and developing a fever. Alarmed by the presence of blood in his feces on the second night, he made the decision to seek medical attention. It is likely that Varun is afflicted with Ulcerative Colitis. To gain a comprehensive understanding of this condition, let us delve into its intricacies.

Ulcerative colitis, a prevalent inflammatory and ulcerative ailment that impacts the mucosal and submucosal layers of the colon is known as a condition. Although it can manifest at any age, it is more frequently observed among the younger population. Typically, the onset of symptoms is gradual.

7.1. Etiology

Despite the absence of a definitive etiological cause, it is widely believed that genetic auto-immune factors play a significant role in the development of this condition. Exacerbations of symptoms are frequently observed in individuals experiencing mental conflict and emotional stress. Additionally, there is a potential association between the onset of the disease and allergies to specific foods, notably milk.

7.2. Clinical symptoms

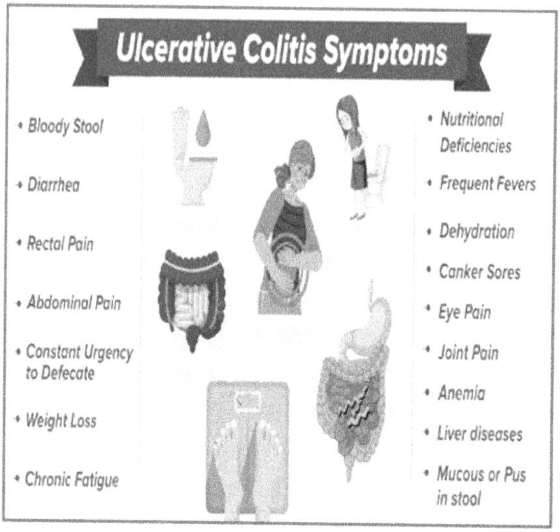

The common symptoms are:

1. The individual experiences mild abdominal discomfort and a frequent urge to defecate multiple times throughout the day.

2. Diarrhea is present along with rectal bleeding.

3. Symptoms include weight loss, dehydration, fever, anemia, and overall weakness.

4. In the early stages, the mucosa appears swollen and inflamed.

5. In more advanced cases, the mucosa undergoes necrosis and develops noticeable ulcers.

7.3. Dietary management

Proper management of diet is crucial in order to maintain the patient's nutritional status. Due to the gradual development of the condition and the lengthy recovery process, long-term care is typically necessary. Now, let us delve into the fundamental aspects of nutritional control.

Dietary control and nutritional recommendations require individualized attention. The tolerance for different meals can vary greatly from one patient to another, depending on the severity of their illness and nutritional issues. The first step is to determine the patient's calorie requirements.

7.3.1. Energy

Calorie intake needs to be increased in order to:

1) Restore and maintain a healthy weight.

2) Compensate for the elevated basal metabolic rate (BMR).

3) Promote growth, particularly in teenagers. It is recommended to consume a daily caloric intake of 40-50 Kcal/kg IBW.

7.3.2. Proteins

Patients suffering from ulcerative colitis experience a significant increase in fecal N2 excretion compared to the normal range. On average, they lose around 4-8 g of fecal N2 per day, whereas a healthy individual excretes only 2 g. In severe cases of ulcerative colitis, this loss can escalate to as much as 20 g of N2 per day, which is equivalent to 125 g of protein. Consequently, the levels of serum albumin, a vital protein in the body, are notably low in these patients.

Proteins play a crucial role in various bodily functions such as tissue synthesis and repair. Moreover, they are essential for compensating for the increased stool losses experienced by ulcerative colitis patients. To counterbalance these losses, it becomes necessary to consume substantial amounts of high-quality protein, approximately 1.5 g per ideal body weight (IBW).

For individuals who have an allergy to milk, it is advisable to focus on alternative sources of protein such as soft meats, fish, poultry, and eggs. These options can provide the necessary protein intake while accommodating their dietary restrictions.

7.3.3. Fats

Normal foods containing fats (invisible or intrinsic fat) are acceptable, however fried meals are not, as they are difficult to digest owing to liver dysfunction. As steatorrhea is common in ulcerative colitis, lipids high in medium chain triglycerides should be ingested. The recommended daily intake of total fat is advised to be maintained at 55-60 g, while the consumption of visible fat should be limited to approximately 25-30 g.

7.3.4. Carbohydrates

They are a readily absorbed source of energy. Bulk-producing veggies are restricted to improve nutrient intake. Sugars and starches can contribute to an increase in calorie intake.

7.3.5. Fiber

Eliminating roughage appears to have a stronger effect on avoiding illness relapses. To avoid serious bleeding during diarrhea, a low residue meal may be administered during an acute bout. Following that, because many ulcerative colitis patients cannot stomach raw vegetables, some degree of fiber restriction is usually required. It has the potential to aggravate the already irritated mucosa. Vegetables can be offered in a variety of formats. All irritating and spicy meals should be avoided at all costs. Raw vegetables, spicy meals, and irritants should be avoided.

7.3.6. Vitamins

Commercial multivitamin supplements, especially those necessary for the recovery process and the metabolism of calories and proteins, ought to be consumed orally.

7.3.7. Mineral

Mineral deficiencies can have serious consequences if left untreated. In the case of a patient with moderately advanced ulcerative colitis, the excessive passing of feces can result in significant salt loss. To address this, it is recommended to increase oral sodium consumption by adding salt to meals. Additionally, potassium loss is estimated to be 30 mEq / 2.2 g potassium chloride per liter of stool. This can lead to symptoms such as weakness, hypotonia, abdominal distension, and even abnormal electrocardiograms. Oral potassium salts, like potassium citrate, can be beneficial in addressing this deficiency.

Furthermore, the absence of milk in the diet may require calcium supplementation of 400-800 mg per day. It is important to maintain a proper protein to calcium ratio for optimal utilization. On the other hand, oral intake of iron is often poorly tolerated. In such cases, a daily administration of 30 mg of elemental iron is recommended. If anemia is present, blood transfusions may be necessary.

7.3.8. Fluids

To avoid dehydration, a large amount of fluid should be consumed. A patient is properly hydrated if he or she passes at least 1200 ml of urine.

8. Short bowel syndrome (SBS)

Short bowel syndrome pertains to a range of complications experienced by individuals who have undergone the removal of at least half of their small intestine. The extensive resection of the digestive tract leads to a decrease in the speed at which feces pass through. Furthermore, any damage inflicted upon the small intestine, specifically the jejunum, hampers the process of nutrient intake and absorption.

Short Bowel Syndrome is a disorder in which nutrients are not effectively absorbed (malabsorption) because of severe intestinal illness or surgical removal of a major part of the small intestine.

Small intestine resection causes diarrhea, fluid and electrolyte abnormalities, and malabsorption, which leads to malnutrition. Gastric motility is improved, especially after ilium resection. The colon gets a heavy load of fluids, electrolytes, and bile salts in this situation, and its ability to absorb salt and water is limited, resulting in diarrhea. The capacity to maintain fluid and electrolyte balance is significantly reduced if the colon is also removed.

If the ilium is removed, nutrient absorption suffers. According to studies, fat and carbohydrate absorption is decreased by up to 50-75% of consumption. Mineral and vitamin absorption is also hampered. The small bowel hypertrophies and enhances its absorptive function throughout time. This is a human body adaptation mechanism.

8.1. Etiology

The disease is caused by various etiological factors, including:

1. Anaemia

2. Osteoporosis

3. Stone formation

4. Reduced susceptibility to infection

5. Dehydration

8.2. Symptoms

Diarrhoea is the main symptom of short bowel syndrome. Other symptoms include:

1. Anorexia
2. Steatorrhea
3. Heart bum and cramping
4. Bloating and abdominal pain

5. Extreme fatigue
6. Weight loss
7. Fluid retention
8. Anemia and osteomalacia

Many patients with short bowel syndrome are malnourished as small intestine is unable to absorb enough water, vitamins, and other nutrients from their diet. They may also get dehydrated, which can be fatal. Weakness, weariness, sadness, weight loss, bacterial infections, and dietary allergies are all symptoms of dehydration and malnutrition.

8.3. Complications

Short bowel syndrome complications primarily arise from malnutrition. Individuals with short bowel syndrome often experience deficiencies in several vital nutrients, such as calcium, folate, iron, magnesium, vitamin B, and zinc.

8.4. Dietary Management

The symptoms described above must indicate that the condition causes lower food intake, poor absorption, and also weight loss. Several nutrients are typically deficient in the patient. As a consequence, the objectives of nutritional management should encompass the following:

- Alleviating symptoms
- Rectifying nutritional deficiencies
- Diminishing inflammation and mitigating pain.

Dietary considerations should aim to supply an adequate amount of calories. In certain cases, specialized feeding methods like enteral and parenteral feeding may be necessary. It is important to bear in mind the following points:

- A diet that is high in calories but low in residue, while also providing essential vitamins, minerals, and other nutrients, is necessary. The meal should lack flavor.
- It is necessary to follow a diet that is both high in calories and low in residue, while also ensuring the intake of vitamins, minerals, and other essential nutrients. The meal should have no taste.
- To meet the requirements, a diet that is high in calories but low in residue, and also contains essential vitamins, minerals, and other nutrients, is essential. The meal should be devoid of any flavor.
- A diet that is low in residue but high in calories, and also includes vital vitamins, minerals, and other nutrients, is mandatory. The meal should be tasteless.
- It is necessary to adhere to a diet that is high in calories but low in residue, while also providing the necessary vitamins, minerals, and other nutrients. The meal should lack any taste.Short Bowel Syndrome is treated with nutritional supplements and dietary restrictions. To maintain optimal tissue function, vitamin and mineral supplements may need to be many times higher than the conventional suggested daily intakes.
- When necessary, special nutrition to be is administered (enteral and parenteral feeding). Oral feedings are initiated with a simple soft meal that can

be digested without much labour in the intestines.The diet's complexity progressively increases over time, allowing the surviving digestive system to adjust. Finally, patients are weaned totally off enteral feeding and obtain all their nourishment through oral consumption of ordinary meals. If parenteral nutrition is required, it can be administered, although enteral nutrition is recommended.

- Drug treatment is used to supplement dietary control. Anti-inflammatories, immunosuppressants, antibiotics, corticosteroids, and antidiarrheal medicines are frequently utilized.

9. Crohn's disease

Crohn's disease is classified as an inflammatory bowel disease (IBD) that induces inflammation of the tissues in the digestive tract, leading to symptoms such as stomach discomfort, severe diarrhea, exhaustion, weight loss, and malnutrition. The inflammation associated with Crohn's disease can affect various parts of the digestive system, with the small intestine being the most commonly affected area. This inflammation can penetrate the deeper layers of the bowel, causing significant pain and debilitation, and in some cases, fatal consequences. Unfortunately, there is currently no known cure for Crohn's disease, but medications can effectively alleviate symptoms and potentially induce long-term remission and inflammatory healing. With proper medication, many patients with Crohn's disease can lead normal lives.

9.1. Causes

The exact cause of Crohn's disease remains uncertain, despite extensive research. While diet and stress were previously believed to be contributing factors, it is now understood that these variables may exacerbate the condition, but do not directly cause it. Rather, the development of Crohn's disease is likely influenced by a combination of factors.

One such factor is the immune system. While it is possible that a virus or bacteria may trigger the onset of Crohn's disease, no definitive evidence has been found to support this theory. Instead, it is believed that an abnormal immune response may prompt the immune system to attack cells in the digestive tract, leading to the development of the disease.

Another potential factor is heredity. Studies have shown that individuals with a family history of Crohn's disease are more likely to develop the condition, suggesting that genetic factors may play a role in its development. However, it is important to note that the majority of Crohn's disease patients do not have a family history of the condition.

In conclusion, while the precise etiology of Crohn's disease remains uncertain, it is believed to be influenced by a combination of factors, including the immune system and genetic predisposition. Further research is needed to fully understand the underlying mechanisms of this complex disease.

9.2. Risk factors

Crohn's disease risk factors may include:

1. **Age:** Crohn's disease can manifest at any age, although it is most commonly observed in young individuals. A significant number of Crohn's disease patients receive their diagnosis before reaching the age of 30.
2. **Ethnicity:** While Crohn's disease can affect individuals of any ethnic background, those of Eastern European (Ashkenazi) Jewish descent, particularly whites, are at the highest risk. However, there is an increasing prevalence of Crohn's disease among Black populations in North America and the United Kingdom. Additionally, Middle Easterners and migrants to the United States are also experiencing a rise in the occurrence of Crohn's disease.
3. **Family History:** Having a first-degree family member, such as a parent, sibling, or child, with Crohn's disease significantly increases one's risk. Approximately one in every five individuals with Crohn's disease has a family member who also suffers from the condition.
4. **Smoking Cigarettes:** Cigarette smoking is the most influential modifiable risk factor for Crohn's disease. Smoking not only exacerbates the severity of the illness but also heightens the likelihood of requiring surgical intervention. It is imperative to cease smoking in order to mitigate these risks.
5. **Nonsteroidal Anti-inflammatory Drugs:** Examples of such drugs include Ibuprofen (Advil, Motrin IB, and others), naproxen sodium (Aleve), diclofenac sodium, and others. While these medications do not directly cause Crohn's disease, they can induce

intestinal inflammation, thereby worsening the symptoms of Crohn's disease.

9.3. Clinical symptoms

Crohn's disease can affect any portion of your small or big intestine. It may consist of many parts or be continuous. Some patients only have the condition in the colon, which is part of the large intestine.

Crohn's disease symptoms can range from moderate to severe. They normally appear gradually, although they can sometimes appear suddenly and without notice. There may also be times when you have no signs or symptoms (remission).

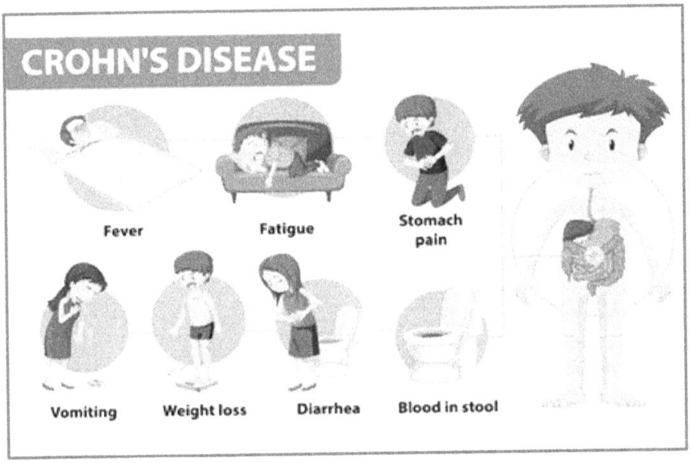

When the disease is active, symptoms typically include:

- Diarrhoea
- Fever
- Fatigue

- Abdominal pain and cramping
- Blood in your stool
- Mouth sores
- Reduced appetite and weight loss
- Pain or drainage near or around the anus due to inflammation from a tunnel into the skin (fistula)

9.4. Other signs and symptoms

Individuals suffering from severe Crohn's disease may also encounter symptoms beyond the confines of the gastrointestinal tract. These symptoms encompass inflammation of the skin, eyes, and joints, as well as inflammation of the liver or bile ducts. Additionally, individuals may experience the formation of kidney stones, iron deficiency leading to anaemia, and in children, delayed growth or sexual development.

9.5. Complications

Crohn's disease may lead to one or more of the following complications:

1. **Obstruction of the bowel:** Crohn's disease possesses the capability to impact the entire thickness of the intestinal wall. Over time, scar tissue forms and constricts sections of the gut, leading to the obstruction of digestive materials. In certain instances, surgical intervention may be necessary to widen the stricture or, in rare cases, remove the affected portion of the intestine.

2. **Ulcers:** Prolonged inflammation can give rise to open sores, known as ulcers, throughout the digestive tract, including the mouth, anus, and genital area (perineum).
3. **Fistulas:** Ulcers can occasionally penetrate the intestinal wall completely, resulting in the formation of a fistula - an abnormal connection between distinct areas of the body. Fistulas can develop between the gut and the skin, as well as between the intestine and another organ. The most common type of fistula is one that occurs in or around the anal region (perianal). The formation of fistulas within the abdominal cavity can lead to the development of infections and abscesses, characterized by the accumulation of pus. If left unattended, these conditions can prove to be fatal. Fistulas may arise between bowel loops, within the bladder or vagina, or penetrate the skin, resulting in the constant discharge of fecal matter onto the skin surface.
4. **Anal Fissure:** An anal fissure refers to a small tear in the tissue surrounding the anus or in the skin around it, which can lead to infection. This condition is often associated with painful bowel movements and may result in the development of a perianal fistula.
5. **Malnutrition:** Diarrhea, gastrointestinal discomfort, and cramping can hinder the ability to consume or absorb sufficient nutrients, leading to malnutrition. Anemia is also common due to low levels of iron or vitamin B-12 caused by the disease.
6. **Colon Cancer:** Individuals with Crohn's disease that affects the colon have an increased risk of developing colon cancer. The standard guidelines for colon

cancer screening recommend a colonoscopy every 10 years for individuals without Crohn's disease, starting at the age of 45. However, for those with Crohn's disease that affects a significant portion of the colon, it is recommended to undergo a colonoscopy approximately 8 years after the disease onset, followed by regular screenings every 1 to 2 years. It is important to consult with your doctor to determine if an earlier or more frequent screening is necessary.

7. **Skin problems:** Numerous people diagnosed with Crohn's disease often experience the emergence of a medical condition known as hidradenitis suppurativa. This condition is characterized by the formation of deep nodules, tunnels, and abscesses in various regions of the body, including the armpits, groin, areas beneath the breasts, and the perianal or vaginal regions.

9.6. Other health issues:

Various other parts of the body can potentially be affected by Crohn's disease. These parts include conditions like low iron levels (anemia), osteoporosis, arthritis, and diseases of the gallbladder or liver. The use of specific medications for Crohn's disease, which work by inhibiting immune system processes, has been linked to an increased risk of developing malignancies such as lymphoma and skin cancer, as well as a higher susceptibility to infections. Moreover, corticosteroids have been associated with a greater incidence of osteoporosis, bone fractures, cataracts, glaucoma, diabetes, and hypertension, among other negative effects. It is recommended to consult a physician to evaluate the potential risks and benefits of medication usage. Additionally, Crohn's disease has been demonstrated to raise the likelihood of blood clots forming in both veins and arteries.

References

1. Irwin H. Rosenberg and Joel B. Mason (1994), Modern Nutrition in health and disease, eight edition, vol: 2, Lea &Febiger, London, pp 1029-1034.

2. Khursheed P. Navder and Charles S. Lieber (2003), Nutritional Aspects and Clinical Management of Chronic Disorders and diseases, CRC press, New Yark .pp- 50-53.

3. Miguel A Gassull and Eduard cabre (2005), Clinical Nutrition, Blackwell publishing company, UK pp 153-156.

4. GBD 2015 Disease and Injury Incidence and Prevalence Collaborators (October 2016). "Global, regional, and national incidence, prevalence, and years lived with disability for 310 diseases and injuries, 1990-2015: a systematic analysis for the Global Burden of Disease Study 2015". Lancet. 388 (10053): 1545–1602. doi:10.1016/S0140-6736(16)31678-6. PMC 5055577. PMID 27733282.

5. GBD 2015 Disease and Injury Incidence and Prevalence Collaborators (October 2016). "Global, regional, and national life expectancy, all-cause mortality, and cause-specific mortality for 249 causes of death, 1980-2015: a systematic analysis for the Global Burden of Disease Study 2015". Lancet. 388 (10053): 1459–1544. doi:10.1016/S0140-6736(16)31012-1. PMC 5388903. PMID 27733281.

6. Talley N (2018). Clinical examination: A systematic guide to physical diagnosis. Chatswood, N.S.W: Elsevier Australia. p. 227. ISBN 978-0-7295-4259-3. OCLC 988941211.

7. Jump up to:a b Baumgart DC, Carding SR (May 2007). "Inflammatory bowel disease: cause and immunobiology". Lancet. 369 (9573): 1627–40. doi:10.1016/S0140-6736(07)60750-8. PMID 17499605. S2CID 13544348.

8. Jump up to:a b Baumgart DC, Sandborn WJ (May 2007). "Inflammatory bowel disease: clinical aspects and established and evolving therapies". Lancet. 369 (9573): 1641–57. doi:10.1016/S0140-6736(07)60751-X. PMID 17499606. S2CID 35264387.

9. Xavier RJ, Podolsky DK (July 2007). "Unravelling the pathogenesis of inflammatory bowel disease". Nature. 448 (7152): 427–34. Bibcode:2007Natur.448..427X. doi:10.1038/nature06005. PMID 17653185. S2CID 4337332.

10. Jump up to:a b c d e f internetmedicin.se >Inflammatorisktarmsjukdom, kronisk, IBD By Robert Löfberg. Retrieved Oct 2010 Translate.

11. Hanauer SB, Sandborn W (March 2001). "Management of Crohn's disease in adults". The American Journal of Gastroenterology. 96 (3): 635–43. doi:10.1111/j.1572-0241.2001.3671_c.x (inactive 1 August 2023). PMID 11280528. S2CID 31219115.

12. Wang GF, Ren JA, Liu S, Chen J, Gu GS, Wang XB, et al. (July 2012). "Clinical characteristics of non-perianal fistulating Crohn's disease in China: a single-center experience of 184 cases". Chinese Medical Journal. 125 (14): 2405–10. PMID 22882911.

13. Stein J, Hartmann F, Dignass AU (November 2010). "Diagnosis and management of iron deficiency anemia in patients with IBD". Nature Reviews. Gastroenterology & Hepatology. 7 (11): 599–610. doi:10.1038/nrgastro.2010.151. PMID 20924367. S2CID 25341683.

14. Liu S, Ren J, Zhao Y, Han G, Hong Z, Yan D, et al. (February 2013). "Nonthyroidal illness syndrome: is it far away from Crohn's disease?". Journal of Clinical Gastroenterology. 47 (2): 153–9. doi:10.1097/MCG.0b013e318254ea8a. PMID 22874844. S2CID 35344744.

15. Warner J (February 22, 2011). Martin LJ (ed.). "Inflammatory Bowel Disease Health Center". WebMD. Retrieved 14 October 2014.

16. Lu DG, Ji XQ, Liu X, Li HJ, Zhang CQ (January 2014). "Pulmonary manifestations of Crohn's disease". World Journal of Gastroenterology. 20 (1): 133–41. doi:10.3748/wjg.v20.i1.133. PMC 3886002. PMID 24415866.

17. Aydoğdu, Müge; Gürsel, Gül; Özyilmaz, Ezgi; Akyürek, Nalan; Memış, Leyla (2012). "A case of ulcerative colitis complicated with bronchiolitis obliterans organizing pneumonia (BOOP) and air leak

syndrome". The Turkish Journal of Gastroenterology. 23 (5): 590–595. doi:10.4318/tjg.2012.0428. ISSN 2148-5607. PMID 23161307.

18. Rubin DT, Ananthakrishnan AN, Siegel CA, Sauer BG, Long MD (March 2019). "ACG Clinical Guideline: Ulcerative Colitis in Adults". The American Journal of Gastroenterology. 114 (3): 384–413. doi:10.14309/ajg.0000000000000152. PMID 30840605. S2CID 73473272.

19. Hanauer SB, Sandborn W (March 2001). "Management of Crohn's disease in adults". The American Journal of Gastroenterology. 96 (3): 635–43. doi:10.1111/j.1572-0241.2001.3671_c.x (inactive 1 August 2023). PMID 11280528. S2CID 31219115.

20. Broomé U, Bergquist A (February 2006). "Primary sclerosing cholangitis, inflammatory bowel disease, and colon cancer". Seminars in Liver Disease. 26 (1): 31–41. doi:10.1055/s-2006-933561. PMID 16496231.

21. Shepherd NA (August 2002). "Granulomas in the diagnosis of intestinal Crohn's disease: a myth exploded?". Histopathology. 41 (2): 166–8. doi:10.1046/j.1365-2559.2002.01441.x. PMID 12147095. S2CID 36907992.

22. Mahadeva U, Martin JP, Patel NK, Price AB (July 2002). "Granulomatous ulcerative colitis: a re-appraisal of the mucosal granuloma in the distinction of Crohn's disease from ulcerative colitis". Histopathology. 41 (1): 50–5. doi:10.1046/j.1365-

2559.2002.01416.x. PMID 12121237. S2CID 29476514.

23. DeRoche TC, Xiao SY, Liu X (August 2014). "Histological evaluation in ulcerative colitis". Gastroenterology Report. 2 (3): 178–92. doi:10.1093/gastro/gou031. PMC 4124271. PMID 24942757.

24. Elson CO, Cong Y, Weaver CT, Schoeb TR, McClanahan TK, Fick RB, Kastelein RA (2007). "Monoclonal anti-interleukin 23 reverses active colitis in a T cell-mediated model in mice". Gastroenterology. 132 (7): 2359–70. doi:10.1053/j.gastro.2007.03.104. PMID 17570211.

25. Ananthakrishnan AN, Kaplan GG, Bernstein CN, Burke KE, Lochhead PJ, Sasson AN, Agrawal M, Tiong JHT, Steinberg J, Kruis W, Steinwurz F, Ahuja V, Ng SC, Rubin DT, Colombel JF, Gearry R; International Organization for Study of Inflammatory Bowel Diseases. Lifestyle, behaviour, and environmental modification for the management of patients with inflammatory bowel diseases: an International Organization for Study of Inflammatory Bowel Diseases consensus. Lancet Gastroenterol Hepatol. 2022 Apr 26:S2468-1253(22)00021-8.

26. Roncoroni L, Gori R, Elli L, Tontini GE, Doneda L, Norsa L, Cuomo M, Lombardo V, Scricciolo A, Caprioli F, Costantino A, Scaramella L, Vecchi M. Nutrition in Patients with Inflammatory Bowel Diseases: A Narrative Review. Nutrients. 2022 Feb 10;14(4):751.

27. Limketkai, Berkeley N.; Hamideh, Mohamed; Shah, Rishabh; Sauk, Jenny S.; Jaffe, Nancee (2022-01-29). "Dietary Patterns and Their Association With Symptoms Activity in Inflammatory Bowel Diseases". Inflammatory Bowel Diseases. 28 (11): 1627–1636. doi:10.1093/ibd/izab335. ISSN 1536-4844. PMID 35092268.

28. Rashvand S, Behrooz M, Samsamikor M, Jacobson K, Hekmatdoost A (June 2018). "Dietary patterns and risk of ulcerative colitis: a case-control study". Journal of Human Nutrition and Dietetics. 31 (3): 408–412. doi:10.1111/jhn.12544. PMID 29468761. S2CID 3452004.

29. Limketkai BN, Sepulveda R, Hing T, Shah ND, Choe M, Limsui D, Shah S (February 2018). "Prevalence and factors associated with gluten sensitivity in inflammatory bowel disease". Scandinavian Journal of Gastroenterology. 53 (2): 147–151. doi:10.1080/00365521.2017.1409364. PMID 29216767. S2CID 4119392.

30. Andersen V, Olsen A, Carbonnel F, Tjønneland A, Vogel U (March 2012). "Diet and risk of inflammatory bowel disease". Digestive and Liver Disease. 44 (3): 185–94. doi:10.1016/j.dld.2011.10.001. PMID 22055893.

31. Barron M (2021-01-11). "Sugar may trigger inflammatory bowel disease by breaking down gut mucus". Massive Science. Retrieved 2021-01-15.

32. Thomas JP, Modos D, Rushbrook SM, Powell N, Korcsmaros T. The Emerging Role of Bile Acids in the Pathogenesis of Inflammatory Bowel Disease. Front Immunol. 2022 Feb 3;13:829525. doi: 10.3389/fimmu.2022.829525. PMID 35185922; PMCID: PMC8850271

33. Mukhopadhya I, Hansen R, El-Omar EM, Hold GL (February 2012). "IBD-what role do Proteobacteria play?". Nature Reviews. Gastroenterology & Hepatology. 9 (4): 219–30. doi:10.1038/nrgastro.2012.14. PMID 22349170. S2CID 24538712.

34. Aroniadis OC, Brandt LJ (January 2013). "Fecal microbiota transplantation: past, present and future". Current Opinion in Gastroenterology. 29 (1): 79–84. doi:10.1097/MOG.0b013e32835a4b3e. PMID 23041678. S2CID 39943619.

35. Kotanko P, Carter M, Levin NW (August 2006). "Intestinal bacterial microflora--a potential source of chronic inflammation in patients with chronic kidney disease". Nephrology, Dialysis, Transplantation. 21 (8): 2057–60. doi:10.1093/ndt/gfl281. PMID 16762961.

36. Ryan, F. J.; Ahern, A. M.; Fitzgerald, R. S.; Laserna-Mendieta, E. J.; Power, E. M.; Clooney, A. G.; O'Donoghue, K. W.; McMurdie, P. J.; Iwai, S.; Crits-Christoph, A.; Sheehan, D. (2020-03-23). "Colonic microbiota is associated with inflammation and host epigenomic alterations in inflammatory bowel disease". Nature Communications. 11 (1): 1512.

Bibcode:2020NatCo..11.1512R. doi:10.1038/s41467-020-15342-5. ISSN 2041-1723. PMC 7089947. PMID 32251296.

37. Clooney, Adam G.; Eckenberger, Julia; Laserna-Mendieta, Emilio; Sexton, Kathryn A.; Bernstein, Matthew T.; Vagianos, Kathy; Sargent, Michael; Ryan, Feargal J.; Moran, Carthage; Sheehan, Donal; Sleator, Roy D. (March 2021). "Ranking microbiome variance in inflammatory bowel disease: a large longitudinal intercontinental study". Gut. 70 (3): 499–510. doi:10.1136/gutjnl-2020-321106. ISSN 1468-3288. PMC 7873428. PMID 32536605.

38. Maloy KJ, Powrie F (June 2011). "Intestinal homeostasis and its breakdown in inflammatory bowel disease". Nature. 474 (7351): 298–306. doi:10.1038/nature10208. PMID 21677746. S2CID 205225483. Archived from the original on 2019-10-29. Retrieved 2019-10-29.

39. Cario E (September 2010). "Toll-like receptors in inflammatory bowel diseases: a decade later". Inflammatory Bowel Diseases. 16 (9): 1583–97. doi:10.1002/ibd.21282. PMC 2958454. PMID 20803699.

40. Coskun M (2014-08-25). "Intestinal epithelium in inflammatory bowel disease". Frontiers in Medicine. 1: 24. doi:10.3389/fmed.2014.00024. PMC 4292184. PMID 25593900.

41. Pereira, Cristiana; Grácio, Daniela; Teixeira, João P.; Magro, Fernando (October 2015). "Oxidative Stress

and DNA Damage: Implications in Inflammatory Bowel Disease". Inflammatory Bowel Diseases. 21 (10): 2403–2417. doi:10.1097/MIB.0000000000000506. PMID 26193347. S2CID 8068289.

42. Ek WE, D'Amato M, Halfvarson J (2014). "The history of genetics in inflammatory bowel disease". Annals of Gastroenterology. 27 (4): 294–303. PMC 4188925. PMID 25331623.

43. Eijsbouts, Chris; Zheng, Tenghao; Kennedy, Nicholas A.; et al. (November 2021). "Genome-wide analysis of 53,400 people with irritable bowel syndrome highlights shared genetic pathways with mood and anxiety disorders". Nature Genetics. 53 (11): 1543–1552. doi:10.1038/s41588-021-00950-8. ISSN 1546-1718. PMC 8571093. PMID 34741163.

44. Liu TC, Stappenbeck TS (May 2016). "Genetics and Pathogenesis of Inflammatory Bowel Disease". Annual Review of Pathology. 11: 127–48. doi:10.1146/annurev-pathol-012615-044152. PMC 3204665. PMID 26907531.

45. Ye BD, McGovern DP (October 2016). "Genetic variation in IBD: progress, clues to pathogenesis and possible clinical utility". Expert Review of Clinical Immunology. 12 (10): 1091–107. doi:10.1080/1744666X.2016.1184972. PMC 5083126. PMID 27156530.

46. Jostins L, Ripke S, Weersma RK, Duerr RH, McGovern DP, Hui KY, et al. (November 2012).

"Host-microbe interactions have shaped the genetic architecture of inflammatory bowel disease". Nature. 491 (7422): 119–24. Bibcode:2012Natur.491..119.. doi:10.1038/nature11582. PMC 3491803. PMID 23128233.

47. Chu H, Khosravi A, Kusumawardhani IP, Kwon AH, Vasconcelos AC, Cunha LD, et al. (May 2016). "Gene-microbiota interactions contribute to the pathogenesis of inflammatory bowel disease". Science. 352 (6289): 1116–20. Bibcode:2016Sci...352.1116C. doi:10.1126/science.aad9948. PMC 4996125. PMID 27230380.

48. Bocchetti M, Ferraro MG, Ricciardiello F, Ottaiano A, Luce A, Cossu AM, et al. (April 2021). "The Role of microRNAs in Development of Colitis-Associated Colorectal Cancer". International Journal of Molecular Sciences. 22 (8): 3967. doi:10.3390/ijms22083967. PMC 8068787. PMID 33921348.

49. Henderson P, Anderson NH, Wilson DC (May 2014). "The diagnostic accuracy of fecal calprotectin during the investigation of suspected pediatric inflammatory bowel disease: a systematic review and meta-analysis". The American Journal of Gastroenterology. 109 (5): 637–45. doi:10.1038/ajg.2013.131. PMID 23670113. S2CID 30604736.

50. Waugh N, Cummins E, Royle P, Kandala NB, Shyangdan D, Arasaradnam R, et al. (November 2013). "Faecal calprotectin testing for differentiating

amongst inflammatory and non-inflammatory bowel diseases: systematic review and economic evaluation". Health Technology Assessment. 17 (55): xv–xix, 1–211. doi:10.3310/hta17550. PMC 4781415. PMID 24286461.

51. Vaos G, Kostakis ID, Zavras N, Chatzemichael A (2013). "The role of calprotectin in pediatric disease". BioMed Research International (Review). 2013: 542363. doi:10.1155/2013/542363. PMC 3794633. PMID 24175291.

52. "Inflammatory Bowel Disease" (PDF). World Gastroenterology Organization. August 2015. Retrieved Mar 13, 2016.

53. Cappello M, Randazzo C, Bravatà I, Licata A, Peralta S, Craxì A, Almasio PL (2014). "Liver Function Test Abnormalities in Patients with Inflammatory Bowel Diseases: A Hospital-based Survey". Clinical Medicine Insights. Gastroenterology. 7: 25–31. doi:10.4137/CGast.S13125. PMC 4069044. PMID 24966712.

54. "IBD Facts". Archived from the original on 2013-02-12. Retrieved 2013-02-13.

55. Levine, Jonathan S.; Burakoff, Robert (2011). "Extraintestinal Manifestations of Inflammatory Bowel Disease". Gastroenterology & Hepatology. 7 (4): 235–241. ISSN 1554-7914. PMC 3127025. PMID 21857821.

56. Glocker EO, Kotlarz D, Boztug K, Gertz EM, Schäffer AA, Noyan F, et al. (November 2009). "Inflammatory

bowel disease and mutations affecting the interleukin-10 receptor". The New England Journal of Medicine. 361 (21): 2033–2045. doi:10.1056/NEJMoa0907206. PMC 2787406. PMID 19890111.

57. Bennike, Tue; Birkelund, Svend; Stensballe, Allan; Andersen, Vibeke (2014-03-28). "Biomarkers in inflammatory bowel diseases: Current status and proteomics identification strategies". World Journal of Gastroenterology. 20 (12): 3231–3244. doi:10.3748/wjg.v20.i12.3231. ISSN 1007-9327. PMC 3964395. PMID 24696607.

58. "Crohn's & Colitis Foundation of America".

59. ^ Yamamoto-Furusho, J. K.; Bosques-Padilla, F.; de-Paula, J.; Galiano, M. T.; Ibañez, P.; Juliao, F.; Kotze, P. G.; Rocha, J. L.; Steinwurz, F.; Veitia, G.; Zaltman, C. (2017-01-01). "Diagnosis and treatment of inflammatory bowel disease: First Latin American Consensus of the Pan American Crohn's and Colitis Organisation". Revista de Gastroenterología de México (English Edition). 82 (1): 46–84. doi:10.1016/j.rgmxen.2016.07.003. ISSN 2255-534X. PMID 27979414.

60. Guindi M, Riddell RH (December 2004). "Indeterminate colitis". Journal of Clinical Pathology. 57 (12): 1233–44. doi:10.1136/jcp.2003.015214. PMC 1770507. PMID 15563659.

61. Guindi, M; Riddell, R H (2004). "Indeterminate colitis". Journal of Clinical Pathology. 57 (12): 1233–

1244. doi:10.1136/jcp.2003.015214. ISSN 0021-9746. PMC 1770507. PMID 15563659.

62. Agabegi ED, Agabegi SS (2008). "Inflammatory bowel disease (IBD)". Step-Up to Medicine (Step-Up Series). Hagerstwon, MD: Lippincott Williams & Wilkins. pp. 152–156. ISBN 0-7817-7153-6.

63. Feller M, Huwiler K, Schoepfer A, Shang A, Furrer H, Egger M (February 2010). "Long-term antibiotic treatment for Crohn's disease: systematic review and meta-analysis of placebo-controlled trials". Clinical Infectious Diseases. 50 (4): 473–80. doi:10.1086/649923. PMID 20067425.

64. Prantera C, Scribano ML (July 2009). "Antibiotics and probiotics in inflammatory bowel disease: why, when, and how". Current Opinion in Gastroenterology. 25 (4): 329–33. doi:10.1097/MOG.0b013e32832b20bf. PMID 19444096.

65. Mowat C, Cole A, Windsor A, Ahmad T, Arnott I, Driscoll R, et al. (May 2011). "Guidelines for the management of inflammatory bowel disease in adults". Gut. 60 (5): 571–607. doi:10.1136/gut.2010.224154. PMID 21464096. S2CID 8269837.

66. "Pouchitis: Symptoms & Causes". Mayo Clinic. 21 December 2018.

67. Karimuddin A, Gilles G. "Surgery for Abdominal/Intestinal Crohn's Disease". Trusted Therapies. Retrieved 19 May 2015.

68. "Inflammatory Bowel Disease". Mayo Clinic. Retrieved November 18, 2022.

69. DiLauro, Steven; Crum-Cianflone, Nancy F. (2010). "Ileitis: When It Is Not Crohn's Disease". Current Gastroenterology Reports. 12 (4): 249–258. doi:10.1007/s11894-010-0112-5. ISSN 1522-8037. PMC 2914216. PMID 20532706.

70. Cohen, Benjamin L.; Torres, Joana; déric Colombel, Jean-Fré (2012). "Immunosuppression in inflammatory bowel disease: how much is too much?". Current Opinion in Gastroenterology. 28 (4): 341–348. doi:10.1097/MOG.0b013e328354567f. ISSN 0267-1379. PMC 6681654. PMID 22573191.

71. D'Haens GR, Panaccione R, Higgins PD, Vermeire S, Gassull M, Chowers Y, et al. (February 2011). "The London Position Statement of the World Congress of Gastroenterology on Biological Therapy for IBD with the European Crohn's and Colitis Organization: when to start, when to stop, which drug to choose, and how to predict response?". The American Journal of Gastroenterology. 106 (2): 199–212, quiz 213. doi:10.1038/ajg.2010.392. PMID 21045814. S2CID 24401720.

2.

Inflammatory Bowel Disease, Its Pathophysiology and Morphology

Mori Hetshi Pravinbhai, Vaghela Archana Gopalbhai, Vasani Ruta Kiritbhai

Student

P P Savani University, Kosamba, Surat

Email: morihetshi10@gmail.com

Abstract

Disease diagnosis is extremely important to treat any disease. Signs and symptoms are only things that can convey the physician what treatment the patient needs. Signs and symptoms help us to understand etiological factor, organ damage, progress of illness and its therapeutic management. With the advancement in pathology subject that deals with the study of diseases at cellular level has brought tremendous revolution in medical science. This article is about pathophysiology and morphology of Inflammatory bowel disease (IBD), that explains minute details of IBD at cellular level with its microscopic picture. In depth information help us to understand whether disease is curable, incurable or palliative. Here types of IBD are discussed with its gross and microscopic changes in detail.

Keywords: Inflammatory bowel disease, Ulcerative Colitis, Crohn's Diseases, Pathology, Morphology

1. Introduction

Inflammatory bowel disease (IBD) is a chronic illness resulting from disturbed interactions between gut flora and immunity of the host in genetically predisposed individuals. Inflammatory bowel disease (IBD) comprises of ulcerative colitis and crohn's disease. The difference between ulcerative colitis and crohn's disease is based on the regions affected and the manifestation of the morphologic changes at these particular regions. Colon and rectum are involved in case of Ulcerative colitis and is restricted to the mucosal and submucosal layers. Whereas lower end of small intestine and initial part of large intestine are involved in case of crohn's disease, typically transmural pattern. Crohn disease is also termed as regional enteritis involving any region of the digestive tract.

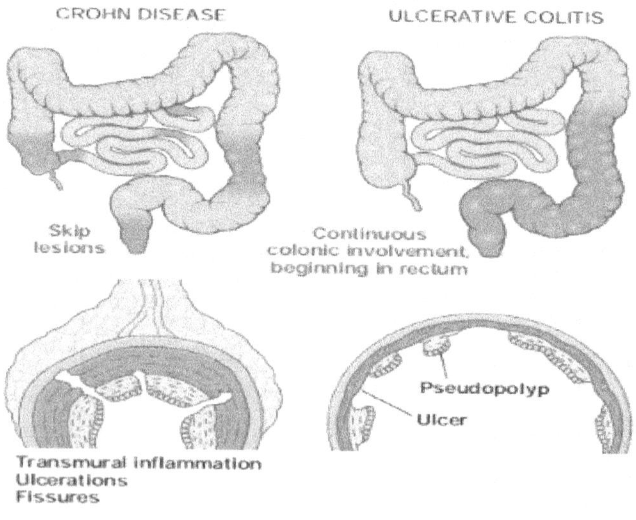

2. Pathogenesis

Polygenic Nature of IBD for which environmental and genetic factors, immunological imbalance, gut barrier permeability and composition of the gut flora play significant role in the pathogenesis of the disease. Though clear mechanism and cause of IBD is not known.

Genetic aspect

Genetic encoding of immune signaling and cytokines are associated with IBD. Genetic polymorphisms in NOD2 is strongly associated with Crohn's disease.

Mucosal immunity

Polymorphism in genes of receptors of both proinflammatory and anti-inflammatory, signaling are involved. Th1 differentiation is seen in both type of diseases, also Th2 activation is observed in ulcerative colitis, this shows differences in genes linked with disease. Crohn disease as well ulcerative colitis both are are associated with polymorphisms in the IL-23 receptor responsible for Th17 signaling. Th17 T-cells are visualised within diseased intestine.

Autophagy and cellular stress responses

ATG16L1 and IRGM genes, responsible for autophagosome formation are defective in autophagy and cellular stress responses leads to IBD. Mechanism of autophagy, clears damaged organelles as well free radicles (ROS) as well intracellular pathogens.

Host-microbial interactions

Microbial products activate receptors like TLRs, dectin and also intracellular microbial-linked pattern receptors, e.g., NOD2. By this mucosal immunity can be modified by the micrbiome. On the other hand, luminal secretion of antimicrobial peptides and antibody IgA significantly alter the gut flora. This interaction between immune system and microbes leads to dysbiosis, characterized by changes in microbial composition with less species diversity.

Crohn's Disease

Also termed as regional enteritis affects any region of the GIT but commonly affects terminal ileum, ileocecal valve, and cecum.

3. Morphology

In about 40% of cases lesions are restricted up to the small intestine; the small intestine and colon are both affected in almost 30% of cases; the rest of the patientsshow involvement of colon only.

Gross pathology

Lesions - Multiple, sharply defined, separate areas, leading to **skip lesions**, are the differentiating feature of crohn's disease from the ulcerative colitis.

Figure - A - Strictures commonly seen in Crohn disease develops as a sequale of inflammatory process, fibrosis (of submucosa), hypertrophy seen in the muscularis propria layer.

Figure - B Aphthous ulcer is the earliest lesion. When multiple lesions often coalesce. patchy distribution of lesion gives cobblestone appearance to the intestinal mucosa

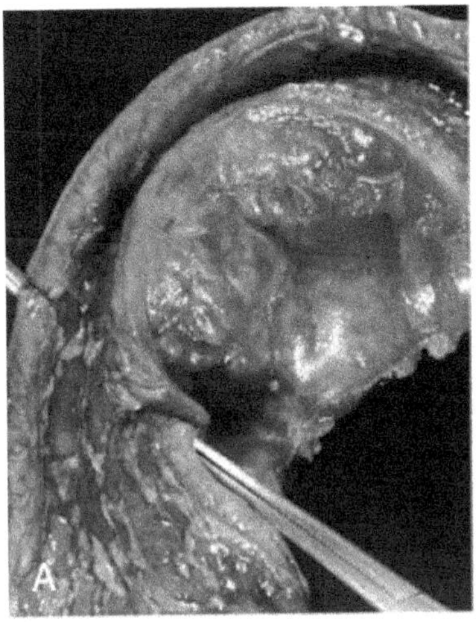

(A) Stricture seen in Small intestine.

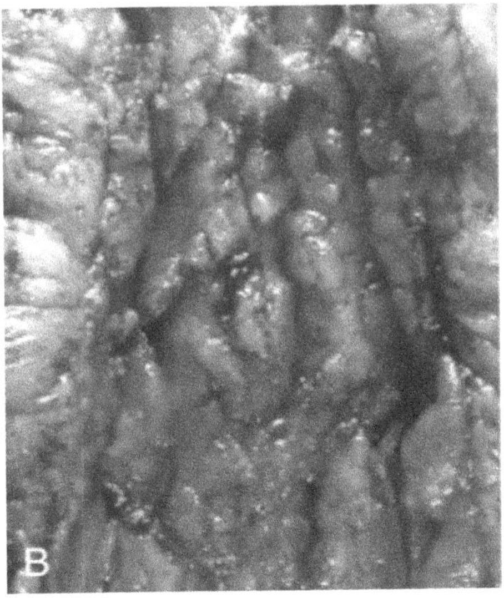

(B) Cobblestone appearance due to ulcer

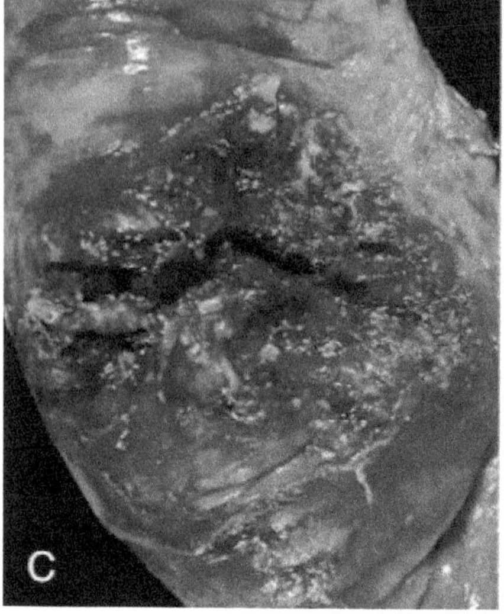

(C) Perforation with serous inflammation

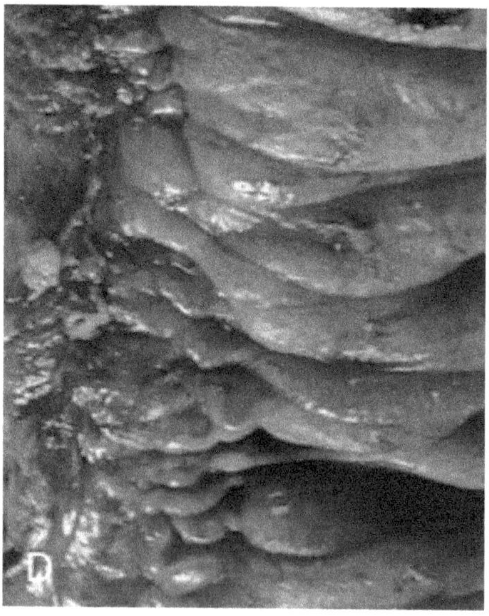

(D) Fatty extensions over the serosal surface.

Figure – c- showng fissures, extending deep to create fistula tracts or perforations.

On account of transmural edema, intestinal wall becomes rubbery and thickened.

Figure - D - Creeping fat is seen in severe transmural disease.

Microscopic features

Crypt epithelium is infiltrated with **numerous neutrophils**. Bunch of neutrophils seen within a crypt epithelium are termed as crypt **abscesses** with damage of crypt epithelium.

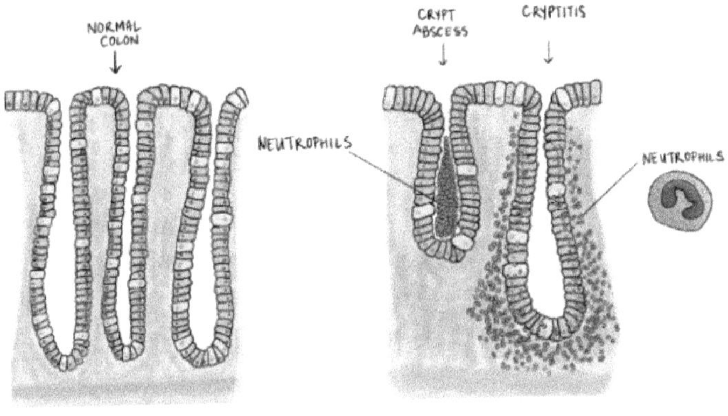

Though grossly it appears as diffuse disease but microscopically shows **patchy ulceration** with random transition between ulcerated and adjacent normal mucosa.

Mucosal glands are distorted and disorganized due to repeated injury and regeneration of crypt epithelium; crypts show bizarre branching shapes (normally straight and parallel) and haphazard crypt organization as shown in figure A.

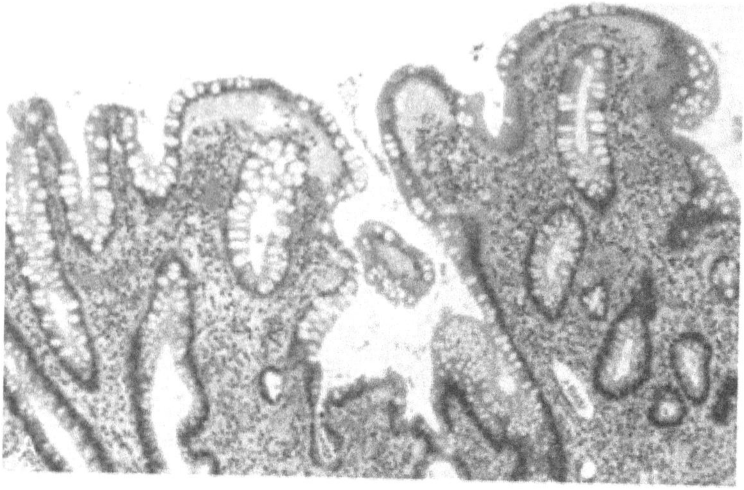

Crypt disorganization resulting from repeated destruction and regeneration eventually leads to epithelial metaplasia. Atrophy of mucosa and destruction of crypts develop after many years. Hallmark of Crohn disease is noncaseating granulomas. (figure - B)

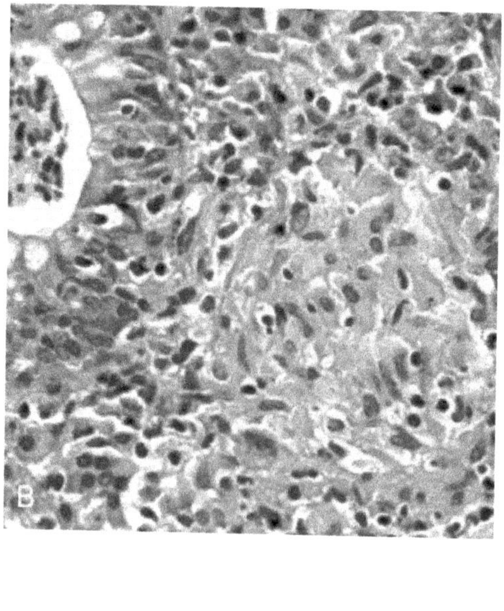

As shown in the picture- C- below- is noncaseating granulomas (seen in active phase of disease in 35% of cases) - with ulceration and purulent exudate.

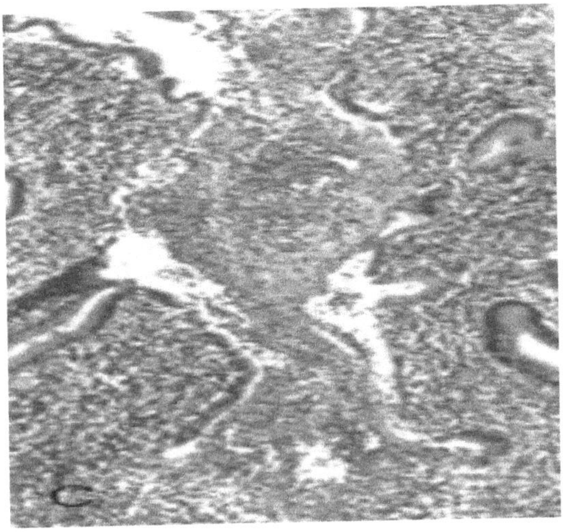

Noncaseating granulomas also appear in uninvolved areas as shown in figure D below (arrows).

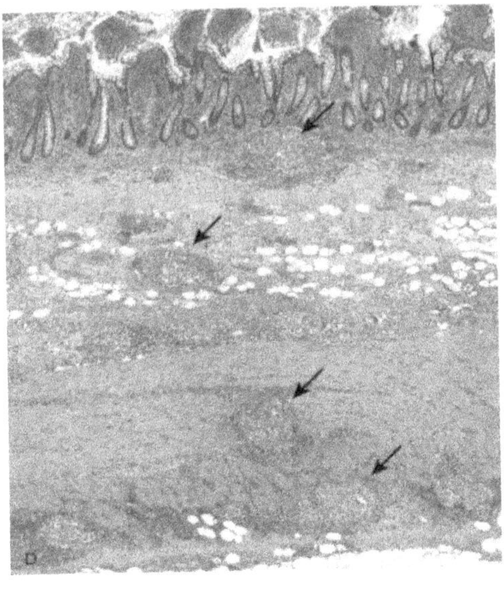

Ulcerative Colitis

Involves mainly the colon and rectum.

Gross pathology

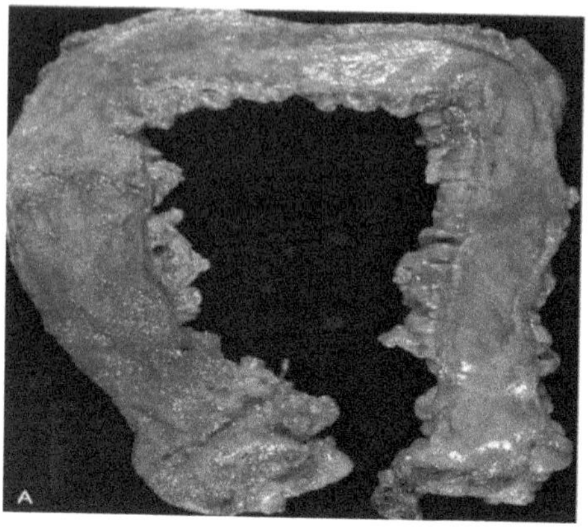

Figure A is showing Pancolitis (active phase disease). Disease involving entire colon is called pancolitis. Inflamed mucosa seen in the cecum on the left and on right side atrophic, smooth mucosa are seen distally.

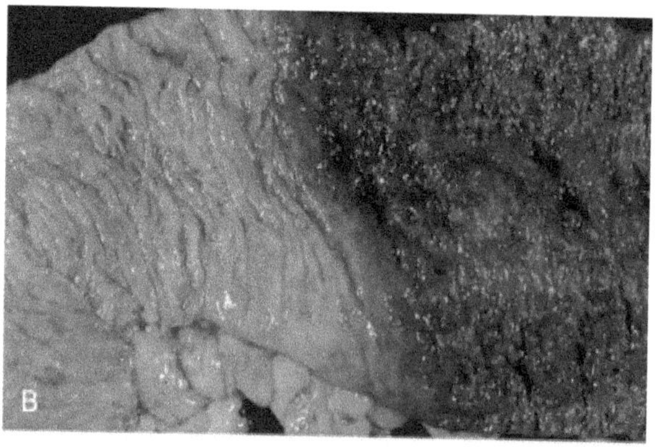

Figure B showing – Clearline of demarcation seen between normal mucosa & active ulcerative colitis on left &right side respectively.

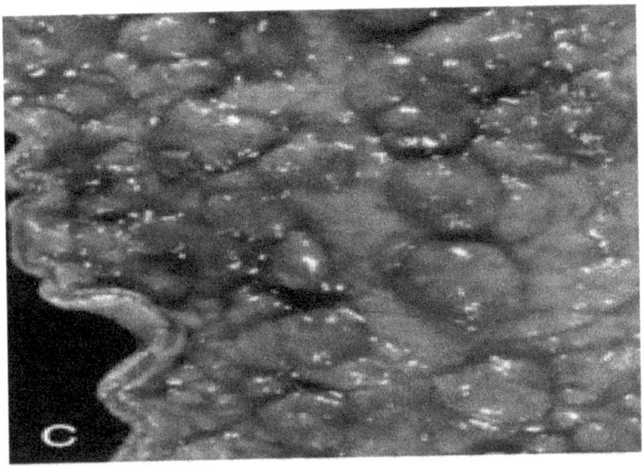

Figure – C shows inflammatory pseudopolyps formed due to regenerating mucosa bulging into the intestinal lumen appearing like polyps

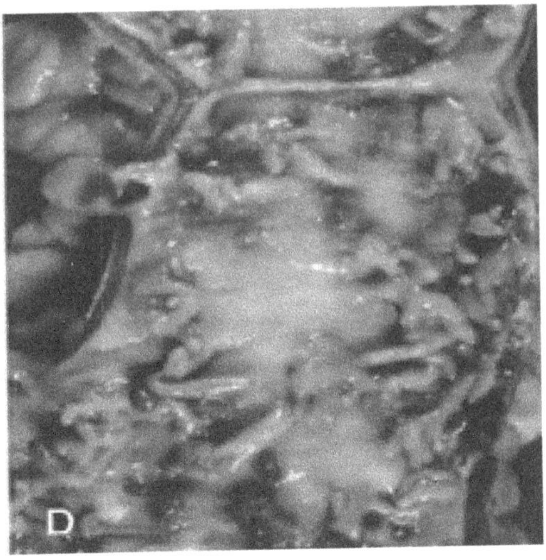

Figure –D – showing mucosal bridges (formed by fusion of the tips of these polyps) can connect inflammatory polyps.

Eventually ulcers begin to appear, in case of chronic condition mucosal atrophy shows lack of normal folds. Rarely, in severe cases show dilation of colon as well toxic megacolon, with the risk of perforation.

Histologic characteristics

Mucosal lesions show infiltration of neutrophils,just like Crohn disease, causing crypt abscesses.

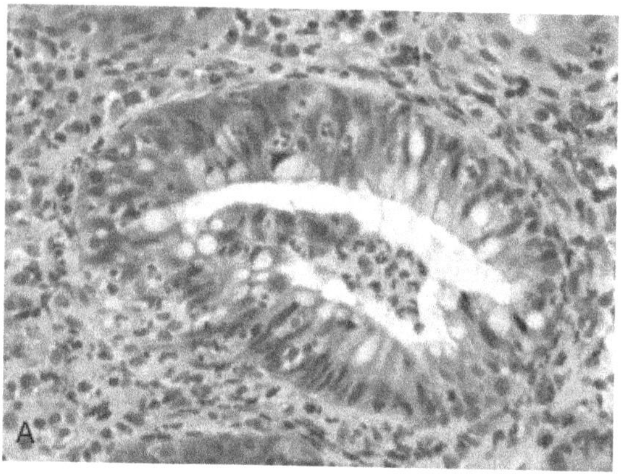

(A) Crypt abscess.

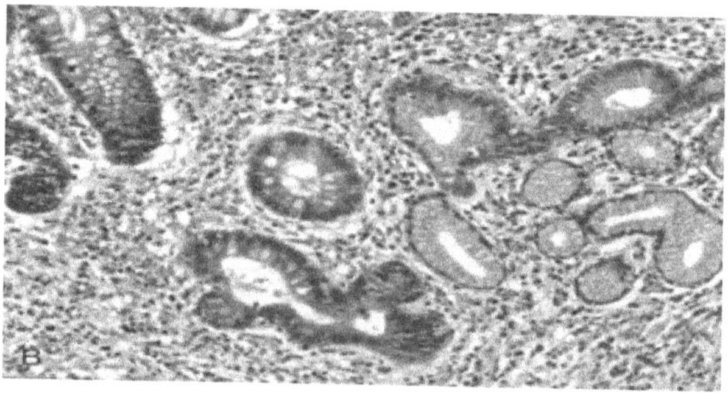

Figure – B showing Pseudopyloric epithelial metaplasia (right) and Crypt distortion.

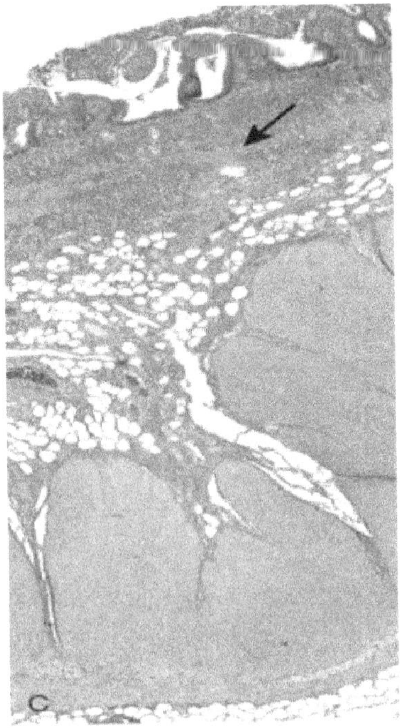

Figure C shows disease is restricted to the mucosal layer (above the arrow).

In severe cases ulcers may penetrate into the submucosal layer sparing muscularis propria. Healing evidences are seen as fibrosis of submucosal layer, atrophy of mucosal layer, and distorted mucosal architecture still histology can revert to almost normal after prolonged remission.

References

1. Kumar, Abbas, Aster, Robbins & Cortan, Pathologic basis of disease,2021,10th edition, Elsevier, p.799-803
2. Mohan Harsh, Text Book of Pathology, Edition 7th, Jaypee Brothers Medical Publishers (P) Ltd, p. 542-545

3. Russell R C G,Bailey & Love's a short practice of surgery, 22 Edition, Chapman & Hall, p.790-798

4. Das. S, A concise Textbook of Surgery with Orthopaedics & Factures, 4th Edition,2006, p.1038-1047

3.

Role of Nosodes in the Treatment of Inflammatory Bowel Disease & Its Dietary Management

Dr. Chetna Rochani, MD (Hom),

PG-FHPC

Consulting Homoeopathic Physician, Vadodara, Gujarat.

Associate Professor & HOD, Department of Pathology

P P Savani University, Kosamba, Surat.

Email: drchetnarochani18@gmail.com

Phone number: +91 8401309348

Dr. Vijaykumar Gopaldas Rajani

BE (Mechanical), D.N.Y.S

Consulting Naturopath, Vadodara, Gujarat

Email: vijayg861@gmail.com

Abstract

To cure any disease, we must understand the evolution & nature of disease in an individual. Inflammatory Bowel Disease includes two bowel diseases; these are (I) Crohn's disease (regional enteritis) and (II) ulcerative colitis. Exact cause is not known yet various infections, immunological mechanism, psychological stress, genetic predisposition, food allergies particularly to milk are considered to be etiological factors. It's always been challenging to cure Inflammatory Bowel Disease. Even if it gets resolved by any means, there are fair chances of relapse. Role of Nosodes in Homoeopathic practice has always been significant in curing chronic conditions like IBD, to complete the cure, prevent the relapses and subsequent attacks, in suppressed and mal treated cases, also used as an intercurrent remedy in genetically predisposed individuals to remove miasmatic block. Nosodes are prescribed on the totality of the patient's symptoms. This paper highlights the importance of different Nosodes as prescription in curing Inflammatory Bowel Disease, its indications, understanding of miasmatic background in depth in different constitutions along with dietary management of the case. As we know the function of intestine is to digest the food, absorb the nutrients and solidify the waste and hence diet plays an important role in weak and defenceless constitutions where dietary corrections are mandatory to remove the obstacle.

Keywords: Nosodes, Inflammatory Bowel Disease, Ulcerative Colitis, Crohn's disease, gastroenterology

1. Introduction

A Nosode is a homoeopathic remedy prepared from an infectious disease product either from the infecting agents like bacteria or virus directly, or less directly from the diseased tissue claimed to contain it. Due to the process of drug dynamisation, disease causing capacity of nosode is lost but its disease curing powers are immensely aroused.

Infecting agents bacterias, viruses being micro sized organismscannot be taken separately for the preparation of medicines and hence nosodes are prepared from diseased products, infected discharges, pustules,diseased tissues like diseased lungs, discharges like sputum, pus, saliva, stool as well cultures of given samples in the laboratory and so on. Nosodes are deeply associated with miasm. Miasm exhibit their infectious nature like infecting agent bacteria, viruses, parasites, fungi etc. and therefore responsible for transmitting disease from one person to another. On other hand miasmcan also be inherited, perceived as the state behind entire totality of symptoms in the given each individual case.

That's why even in the absence of anymicroorganism Homeopathy can still definitely take care of the residual effects of the infection. Conventional mode of treatment is absolutely helpless, unless anduntilan infective agent is present, in such condition either it palliate or suppress the phenomenon more towards deeper layers. It is seen that majority of chronic illnessescould be associated with infective organisms.

In any infective disease condition, material aspect of the disease can be visualised with the aid of microscope whereas the energetic phenomenon remains invisible. It is believed that there is subtle shift in this energetic phenomenon as well in the host may beobserved simultaneously with, or even much prior to the appearance of any illness (includingan infection). This subtle shift in the energetic phenomenon can be perceived by keen observation to the disposition of an individual rather than just identifying the common infective organism. *Disposition of an* *individual,*plays pivotal role for the selection of homeopathic similimum, mainly in the cases spoiled with over drugging, suppression or palliation of the pathological symptoms and paucity of characteristic symptoms of an individual. Consideration of past medical history, family history, nature of an individual, his fears, hobbies, likes, dislikesincluding various aspects of his life *as well as* a specific external etiological factor is mandatory for prescribing a similimum.

These energetic shifts, which act as pre-cursory fields for illness, are termed as*miasms,* and to treat these disturbed dynamic phenomenon, remedies are prepared from actual infective organisms, from discharges or diseased tissues known as *nosodes.*Nosodes treat these dynamic energetic disturbances with a *similar* energetic vibration in an individual.

Dr.Hahneman recognised that remedy is prescribed on the basis of totality of the symptoms, only by knowing pathology cannot really help.Existing dominant miasm must be covered in each individual case. These are known as the true pathognomonic symptoms of the disease. Nosode acts as a constitutional simillimum when administered by the totality of the symptoms just like the mineral, animal and plant remedies.

The mucosal surface of human gastrointestinal tract is about $300m^2$ and is colonised by 10^{13}-10^{14} bacteria consisting of hundreds differentspecies. Colonisation of digestive tract of new born baby begins immediately after the birth and within few days it is completed. Colonisation pattern is affected by mode of delivery and type of diet. Thus, initial colonisation is responsible for designing the final composition of permanent gut flora in adults. This Composition of individual's flora can alter under various conditions, such as diarrhoeal illnesses, drugging with antibiotics, and to some extent triggered by dietary interventions.

Patients seek dietary consultation. Changes in the composition of gut flora plays an important role in the pathogenesis of IBD, to overcome this condition, anti-inflammatory diet (AID) is utilised for case management along with medications.

2. IBD-AID is based on following components:

(1) Restricting certain carbohydrates likelactose, processed or refined complex carbohydrates

(2) Balancing intestinal florawith the help of prebiotics, probiotics likeleek, onions, fiber andfermented food

(3) Increasing intake of omega-3 rich foods and limiting saturated fatty acids intake

(4) Assess of overall dietary habits, digestion and assimilation, identification of individual's intolerance and any nutritional deficiency

(5) Modifying consistency as well texture of the food for better absorption & assimilation, for e.g. cooked, ground, homogenized.

3. Indications of Nosodes

1. Nosode acts as a CONSTITUTIONAL REMEDY when administered on the characteristics mental as well

physical generals and particular symptoms of an individual. For example, Syphilinum in an individual who fears the night because it worsens the sufferings, fear of insanity.Patient has delusions that he isimpure, dirty or tainted, this compels him to wash thehands repeatedly and compulsively. Despairs of the recovery, etc.These symptoms confirm both indicated simillimum remedy as well as the miasmic diagnosis.

2. When WELL SELECTED REMEDIES FAIL TO ACT, PAUSE, OR JUST BRING LITTLE ALTERATION IN THE SYMPTOMS. This generally happens because of the chronic miasms such as psora, sycosis, tubercular and syphilis.

   For example, nosode Tuberculinum, its keynotes are as follow: restlessness, constantly changing symptomatology, and well-selected remedies do not help further, individuals with narrow chest, light complexion, beautiful eyelashes, bright nails, red lips, low vitality and catch cold easily. Dissatisfied, discontented state of mind, aggressive, destructive with a tendency to swear, curse, etc. Fear of animalsspecially dogs, and in general, a desire to travel.

   Another exmaple of nosode Psorinum, its keynotes are: Lack of vital reaction; when well-selected remedies fail to act, in the individuals who are extremely sensitive to cold, their skin appears dirty, with profuse perspiration, filthy odor,hopeless of recovery, etc.

3. When there is PAUCITY OF SYMPTOMS. In case of one-sided diseases, ability of the constitution to manifest the symptoms is repressed by a strong inherited or acquired Miasms.

4. "THE NEVER WELL SINCE SYNDROME", When the individual fail to recover from miasmic infection, and its suppression. For e.g. Medorrhinum, with past history of suppressed gonorrhoea from which patient has never recovered. Probably a new layer of illness has been added.Suppression of gonorrhoea leads to alteration of both mental and physical health. Hence symptoms of a constitutional remedy cannot be manifested on account of the acquired miasm that has become the dominant layer and has suppressed theoriginal basic temperament.

5. WHEN NO ONE REMEDY COMPLETELY FITS THE CASE JUST THE PARTIAL PICTURE OF THE CONSTITUTIONAL REMEDIES ARE MANIFESTED, in this case prescription of a Nosode is needed.

6. WHEN THE PROGRESS OF AN INDICATED CONSTITUTIONAL REMEDY IS HINDERED BY A MIASMIC LAYER. At this junction prescribed nosode is known as intercurrent remedy.

7. Nosode can be used as TO THE DISEASE GENUS. For example, Clark's Pertussin against whooping cough. In the case of adverse effects caused by vaccinesIsodes can be used. In such cases a nosode of that particular vaccination helps to extinguish the adverse-effects of vaccination.

8. Nosode is also used as HOMOEOPATHIC PROPHYLAXIS to prevent specific infectious diseases. For e.g. Variolinum was used to prevent smallpox by Dr.Boenninghausen. Nosodes can protect children from the miasma, inherited through their parents. Dr.J.T.Kent mentioned in his Lectures on Homoeopathic Materia Medica: " All children and young people who have inherited tuberculosis may be immune from their inheritance and their resiliency will be restored if Tuberculinum Bovinum be given in 10m, 50m, Cm. potencies two doses of each potency at long intervals." Thisis mainly related to those children who are extremely nervous, showing temper tantrums, emaciation, swollen glands, frequent colds and anemia like traits of Tubercular Miasm.

9. AUTO-NOSODE. Once Dr.Hahnemannprepared an auto-nosode from the saliva of the patient, suffering from phthisis who was not responding to well-selected remedies.

4. Some Important Nosodes with its indications

1. Pyrogen

This nosode is prepared from septic pus or from decomposed lean beef. Therefore, it is indicated for septic conditions where BLOOD is disorganised. All the dischargesare horribly foul. SORE andBRUISED feeling all over the body.Bed feels very hard. Lymphangitis. Bony pains. History of Recurrent abscesses with violent burning pains. Chronic complaints since suffered from septic conditions;ptomaine poisoning; dissecting wounds, sewer-gas poisoning, remote effects of typhoid fever; chronic malaria, diphtheria, puerperal fever; after effects of miscarriage; where the indicated remedy fails to relieve especially in latent pyogenic processes. Talks or whispers to herself; in sleep.Anxiety and restlessness. Tongue large and flabby, fiery red; brown streak down the centre.Breath horribly offensive.Nausea better by very hot drinks. Thirst for small quantity of cold water, but the least liquid is vomited as soon as it becomes warm.Horribly offensive, brown, black coloured painless, involuntary stool. Complete inertia of rectum.

2. Tuberculinum [Tub.]

This nosode is prepared either from pure cultivation of Mycobacterium tubercule bacilli or from tubercular abscess. Constantly changing symptomatology - complaints appearing suddenly, ceasing suddenly; or even when indicated prescriptionultimately fails to act. Very susceptible to atmospheric changes. Relapsing states. Prostration with good appetite. Susceptible to cold on slightest exposure; leading to diarrhoea. Always feels tired; exertion causes fatigue.Best suited to narrow chested subjects with light complexion. Dissatisfied; desire to travel; cannot remain in one place for long, always desire a change, always wish to do something different.Reckless. Aversion to mental work. Use foul language, curse and swear. Fear of animals specially of dogs. Whines with very little ailments. Craves sweets or cold milk. Aversion to meat. Sudden diarrhoea early in the morning. Watery; black, brown; foul smelling stool; passed with much force. Enlarged lymph nodes. Children suffer from diarrhoea lasting for weeks;

with bluish pallor wasting; and prostration. Inguinal glands indurated and firm. Chronic diarrhoea, with profuse sweat.

3. Baccillus dysenteriae [Dys-co.]

Dysentry Co is the bowel nosode – Shigella dysenteriae and the key note of its use is nervous tension, described as anticipatory anxiety felt before attending an important engagement or before examination. Fear without any apparent reason. Fear of closed places like lifts, train, planes, automobiles, buses etc. Afraid of going out for meeting unknown people. Nervous stammering. Tics of the face. Restless, embarrassed, nervous, depressed. Incapable of struggle, to impose himself.Lips are dry with cracks and fissures. Desire for fatty food, sweetened foods, salty foods, milk. Bad taste in the mouth. Tongue as if scorched. Distended abdomen with flatulence, uneasiness after meals. Pain in the stomach between midnight and 1a. m., better by vomiting of mucus in large quantity. Diarrhoea, frequent stools. Nervous diarrhoea. Sensation of a plug in the rectum, sensation of throbbing in the rectum.

4. Enterococcinum

Digestive system is the primary seat of action of this drug. Tongue white as milk, nausea and anorexia, flatulence, eructations and flatulence is marked. Colitis and enterocolitis which keeps relapsing due to allergic condition.Stools like "cowdung".Morning diarrhoea with great urgency of many stools between 4 to 9 AM. Emotional diarrhoea with profuse mucus.Menstrual diarrhoea.Pain in the colon. Rectal tenesmus.Glairy mucous, bloody diarrhoea.

5. Dietary advice

In General	IBD Meals or snacks to be takenin smaller quantity at more frequent intervals (at 3 or 4 hours interval)
Dietary fiber	IBD 1. Intake of fiber like whole-grains, nuts, seeds and green leafy vegetables should be decreased the during a disease 2. Slowly reintroduce high-fiber foods in small quantity as well one at a time when there no symptoms.
Milk &Milk Products	IBD Restrict milk and dairy based foodsif patient is unable to digest dairy products well, or show lactose intolerance
Fruits & Vegetables	IBD Gas-producing vegetables such as broccoli, cauliflower, cabbage to be avoided that are when the disease is active. Duringdisease flare, peeled vegetables and fruits are recommended.
Carbohydrates	IBD Reducing dietary monosaccharides, disaccharides, and fermentable oligosaccharides help in reducing

	symptoms of IBD.
Lipids	IBD 1. Intake of oils intake should be restricted up to 8 teaspoons per day or even less than that. 2. If patients have loose stool or flatulence, reduce the intake of fatty as well fried foods
Proteins	IBD 1. Lean source of protein such as eggs, fish, tofu or chickencan be more tolerable. 2. Highly processed or fatty, greasy meats should be avoided, such as such as nuggets, sausages,
Beverages	IBD 1. Avoid dehydration. 2. When the disease is active, sweet juices, high sugary drinks, alcohol and caffeine should be avoided.
Dietary supplements	IBD 1. In case of iron deficiency anemia, iron supplementation is recommended. 2. Vitamin D supplementation and Calcium are advised for those patients who are on steroid treatment.

	CD 1. In those cases where more than 20 cm distal ileum is been resected, vitamin B12 supplementation is strongly recommended.
Probiotics	IBD Food must include probiotics and prebiotics.

References

1. Klein Louis, MIASMS AND NOSODES, ORIGINS OF DISEASE, Narayana Verlag, P.5,9,10,12
2. Julian O.A, Julian's Materia Medica of Nosodes with Repertory, B.Jain Publisher (P) LTD, second revised edition, 1985, 15th impression 2020, p.247,248, 574-378,
3. Boericke William, New manual of homoeopathic materia Medica & Repertory, B Jain Publishers Pvt Ltd. 2001, p.1153,1154
4. Allen H.C, Allen's Keynotes and Characteristics with with Nosodes, B. Jain Publishers Pvt. Ltd, 2002, P. 395
5. Phatak S.R., Materia Medica of Homeopathic Medicines, IBPP, 2011, p.602-604, p.491-493
6. Allen J.H, The chronic miasms Psora and pseudopsora, B Jain Publishers Pvt Ltd., 1989, p.58,59

7. Nayak Chaturbuja, Nayak Debadatta, Roja Varanasi, An update on bowel nosode with comparison, B. Jain Publishers Pvt. Ltd, 2015, p.3,6

8. Galande B Tilottama (March 2021), Nosodes and Their Indications in Homoeopathy, *International Journal of Advanced Research in Science, Communication and Technology (IJARSCT),Volume 3,* (Issue 2), p.177-180, DOI: 10.48175/IJARSCT-891

9. Nor Hamizah Shafiee1 , Zahara Abdul Manaf2 , Norfilza M. Mokhtar3,4, Raja Affendi Raja Ali4, Anti-inflammatory diet and inflammatory bowel disease: what clinicians and patients should know?, Intestinal Reasearch, pISSN 1598-9100 • eISSN 2288-1956 https://doi.org/10.5217/ir.2020.00035 Intest Res 2021;19(2):171-185, p.172

Acknowledgement

To the best of our knowledge and belief, it contains no material previously published or written by another person nor does it include contents that are falsified or fabricated. We also sought permission from the copyright owner to use text, illustrations, and/or framework substantively used in the paper.

4.

Curative Treatment of Inflammatory Bowel Disease by Allopathy

Dr. Praveen Katiyar & Ms. Shailendri Kushwaha

Assistant Professor, School of Health Science, CSJM University Kanpur

Ph.D. Scholar, School of Health Science, CSJM University Kanpur

Email: dr.sk7077@gmail.com

Abstract

Inflammatory Bowel Disease (IBD), comprising Crohn's disease and ulcerative colitis, poses a complex challenge involving chronic inflammation of the gastrointestinal tract. Allopathic treatments, though lacking a definitive cure, focus on comprehensive management strategies. Medications such as corticosteroids, 5-aminosalicylic acids, and immunosuppressants play a pivotal role in alleviating symptoms and controlling inflammation. Alongside pharmacological interventions, lifestyle adjustments, including dietary modifications and probiotic use, contribute to symptom relief. In instances of severe disease progression, surgical interventions such as colectomy or strictureplasty become imperative. Post-surgical care involves nuanced medication regimens, nutritional support, diligent monitoring, lifestyle modifications, and psychological assistance. This holistic approach within allopathy underscores the importance of personalized and collaborative strategies to enhance the quality of life for individuals navigating the complexities of IBD.

Key words: Crohn's disease, inflammatory bowel disease, treatment, ulcerative colitis.

1. Introduction

Inflammatory bowel disease (IBD) is also known as Irritable bowel disease. A group of diseases characterized as chronic inflammation and ongoing activation of the immune system and gastrointestinal tract. It is an autoimmune disease which means the body's immune system directly attacks healthy tissues. Inflammatory bowel disease is a complex disorder with various causes that are genetic, immune system dysfunction and environmental factors. The cause of IBD is still unknown, but many researchers suggest that in people with conditions where body's immune system may perceive contaminated food and water, bacteria, viruses and other chemical substances in the intestine as a threat. These conditions cause inflammatory changes, pain, and damages directly to the gastrointestinal track, leading to symptoms like diarrhoea (intestinal infection affecting severely bowel and bladder function leading to abdominal pain, weight loss, and fatigue). Treatment typically involves medication to control inflammation and in some cases surgery to remove damaged portions of the intestines. Inflammatory bowel disease (IBD) hence, has a severe impact on day-to-day life be it education, work or social relationship. It is essential for individual bid IBD to work closely with healthcare providers to manage their condition and maintain a good quality of life. In response, the immune system sends white blood cells to the intestine which causes inflammation. These are directly be cause of stomach pain and many symptoms.

2. Types of Inflammatory bowel disease

The two main types of IBD, Crohn's disease (CD) and ulcerative colitis disease (UD).

2.1. Crohn's disease

Crohn's disease is a chronic inflammatory bowel disease that can affect any part of gastrointestinal tract of the intestine. It makes an impact on the end portions of small intestine is called the ileum, and the beginning of the colon, or large intestine are affected. Crohn's disease affects the entire thickening of intestine wall and may spread other parts of abdomen. It is characterized by inflammation that can spread deep into the layers of the affected intestinal tissues and walls. In this inflammation may cause multiple lesions of the wall of intestines. Many people have severe Crohn's disease, which may result in fistulas or ulcers that form tunnels through the intestinal wall connected to organs. These fistulas may connect several parts of the intestines or the intestine and other organs such as bladder or skin. Which disease may cause scarring in the wall of intestine. which may get narrowed intestinal wall and may cause an obstructions is directly leading to constipation or severe stomach pain. mostly people might be experience irregular cramps and mutable movement of bowel for prolonged period of many years.

Whenever the symptoms of IBD worsen, they usually include one or more symptoms are as followed: persistent diarrhoea and bloody stool, abdominal pain with cramps, constipation, loss of appetite, fatigue, and sudden weight loss. When the inflammatory response causes gastrointestinal symptoms that brings inflammatory changes and severely affects many parts of the human body. Some patients may experience symptoms that seem unrelated to Crohn's disease. In IBD can lead numerous signs and symptoms include mouth sores, skin rashes and lesions, mild fever, arthritis, inflammations in the eyes.

2.2. Ulcerative colitis

Ulcerative colitis (UC) is a chronic inflammatory bowel disease which basically affects the intestinal parts like colon and rectum. However, affect the large intestine wall or colons. Ulcerative colitis causes multiple ulcers in the intestines and infect the mucosal wall of the intestine.

Most commonly ulcerative colitis affects the last end of large intestine especially closest to rectum. There are many symptoms that appear immediately which include irregular bowel movement, frequent diarrhoea and rectal bleeding (bloody stool) with abdominal pain and cramps. Therefore, ulcerative colitis is caused by an abnormal immune system response, people may also experience a loss of appetite, unexpected weight loss, fatigue, skin rashes, and arthritis. Ulcerative colitis is a chronic condition, but symptoms may come and go in changeable patterns.

It is treated with salicylic acid compounds, corticosteroids, immunosuppressive medications and surgeries etc.

3. Curative treatment of IBD using allopathy

Crohn's disease and ulcerative colitis, both conditions of inflammatory bowel disease are typically managed with allopathic or conventional medical treatments. In critical conditions, an affected part of the intestine can be removed by surgery. Curative treatment for IBD is currently not available through allopathy but the aim is to control symptoms include remission and improve the patient's quality of life. IBD symptoms including abdominal pain, diarrhea, bleeding can be reduced and controlled with effective medications. Common treatments include:

3.1. Medication for inflammatory bowel disease

1. Corticosteroid medications- Corticosteroid medications are effective medicine of anti-inflammatory drug and are often used short term to relief symptoms immediately. Corticosteroids such as prednisone or budesonide are often used in short term to control inflammation and manage symptoms of inflammatory bowel disease (IBD). These corticosteroids are given by mouth and as an anima or through intravenous (IV) injections.
2. 5- Amino salicylic Acid specifics - Mainly physicians prescribed 5-aminosalicylic acid specifics is also known as 5-ASAs. Mainly People are affected with inflammatory bowel disease mild to severe. 5-Aminosalicylic Acid are instant effective in ulcerative colitis but sometimes it can also be given in Crohn's disease.

3. They are considered safer for long-term use compared to corticosteroids. These medicines help in reducing intestinal inflammation and wall of the intestine with comfort in stomach pain, diarrhoea with many symptoms. These can be administered orally or through rectal formulations.
4. Immunosuppressive medications- These immunomodulators medication suppress or regulate certain aspects of the immune system, Counteracting the body's abnormal response to food and bacteria in the digestive tract. Physicians may prescribe these medications for long-term use in people with mild or moderate IBD.

3.2. Lifestyle and dietary modifications

Some patients may need to make dietary and lifestyle changes to reduce symptoms and improve overall health. Dietary management for IBD which may include both condition like Crohn's disease and ulcerative colitis can be complex and should be tailored do an individual's specific needs here are some general guidelines.

1. Consulting healthcare professional- Always consult with gastroenterologist or dietitian who is specialized in IBD. They can provide personalized advice based on your specific condition and need.
2. Low residue diet- During a flare-up, lower residue diet, which foods that are high in fiber can relieve burning sensation in the gut.
3. Elemental diet- In severe cases, an elemental diet consisting of pre-digested nutrients may be

recommended to provide nourishment while resting the digestive tract.

4. Anti-inflammatory foods- Incorporate foods rich in omega-3 fatty acids (fatty fish, flaxseeds), antioxidants (fruits and vegetables), and ginger or turmeric, which have anti-inflammatory properties.
5. Small, frequent meals- Eating smaller meals more frequently can help reduce strain on the digestive system.
6. Probiotics- Some individuals with IBD may benefit from probiotics to support gut health.
7. Hydration- Stay well-hydrated to prevent dehydration, which can be a concern with diarrhoea and IBD symptoms.
8. Monitor vitamins and minerals- IBD can lead to nutrient deficiencies, so work with a healthcare professional to ensure you're getting adequate vitamins and minerals, possibly through supplements.
9. Individualized approach- Since IBD affects individuals differently, it's important to tailor your diet to your specific condition and response to different foods.

Always remember that dietary management for IBD is highly individual. Always work closely with a healthcare provider to create a plan that meets your specific needs and helps manage your condition effectively.

3.3. Surgery

In severe cases of IBD surgery to remove damaged portions of the digestive tract although this is not a cure for IBD.

Surgery is an option for individuals with Inflammatory Bowel Disease (IBD) in certain situations. The specific surgical procedures depend on the type of IBD. (Crohn's disease or ulcerative colitis), the location of inflammation, and the patient's individual circumstances. Here are some common surgeries for IBD.

1. Colectomy- This surgery involves the removal of the colon and is typically performed for severe ulcerative colitis when medical treatment is ineffective.
2. Ileostomy- In cases of ulcerative colitis, where the entire colon is removed, an ileostomy may be created. This involves bringing the end of the small intestine (ileum) to the abdominal surface to create a stoma for waste elimination.
3. Colostomy- In some cases of Crohn's disease, when a portion of the colon needs to be removed, a colostomy may be created. This diverts part of the colon to the abdominal surface.
4. Strictureplasty- For Crohn's disease, if there are strictures or narrowing of the small intestine, a strictureplasty may be performed to widen the narrowed area.
5. Resection- In Crohn's disease, when there are localized areas of inflammation and damage, a resection may be performed to remove the affected segment of the intestine.
6. Abscess drainage- In cases where an abscess forms due to infection in the abdominal cavity, surgical drainage may be necessary.

7. Fistula repair- If there are fistulas (abnormal connections between parts of the intestine or between the intestine and other organs), surgical repair may be needed.
8. J-Pouch surgery- For some patients with ulcerative colitis, especially when the entire colon is removed, a J-pouch or ileal pouch-anal anastomosis (IPAA) surgery may be performed. This creates a pouch from the small intestine that is attached to the anal canal, allowing for more normal bowel movements.

The decision to undergo surgery for IBD is typically made based on factors like the severity of the disease, the failure of medical management, and the patient's overall health. It's crucial for individuals with IBD to discuss their options with a healthcare team, including a gastroenterologist and a colorectal surgeon, to determine the most appropriate surgical approach if needed.

4. Symptoms management

Allopathic medicine focus on alleviating symptoms such as abdominal pain, diarrhoea and rectal bleeding through various treatments.

1. Abdominal pain- Crampy abdominal pain is a common symptom of IBD.
2. Diarrhoea- Frequent, loose, or watery stools that occur more frequently than usual.
3. Blood in stool- Rectal bleeding can occur in ulcerative colitis.
4. Weight loss- Due to reduced appetite and malabsorption.
5. Fatigue- IBD can cause chronic fatigue.

6. Fever- Occurs during flares of the disease.
7. Joint pain- Arthritis or joint pain can be associated with IBD.
8. Skin problems- Conditions like erythema nodosum or pyoderma gangrenosum.
9. Mouth sores- Ulcers in the mouth can develop.

6. Surgical treatment of inflammatory bowel disease

Surgical treatment of Inflammatory Bowel Disease (IBD), which includes Crohn's disease and ulcerative colitis, is considered when medical therapies are no longer effective, or when there are complications that require surgical intervention. Here are common surgical procedures for IBD.

1. Colectomy- In cases of severe ulcerative colitis, a colectomy (removal of the colon) may be performed. Depending on the specific procedure, this could result in either an ileostomy (an opening in the abdominal wall through which waste exits the body) or an ileoanal pouch procedure (creation of an internal pouch to collect stool).
2. Resection- In Crohn's disease, segments of the diseased bowel may be removed in a procedure known as a resection. The healthy portions of the intestine are then reconnected.
3. Strictureplasty- This procedure is used to widen narrowed sections of the bowel without removing any part of it. It's often used in Crohn's disease to address strictures.
4. Temporary Ostomies- In some cases, a temporary ileostomy or colostomy may be created to allow the

bowel to rest and heal after surgery. These can later be reversed in a second procedure.

5. Fistula or Abscess Treatment- Surgical intervention may be required to drain and repair fistulas or abscesses that can develop as complications of Inflammation of bowel disease.
6. Colectomy with Ileorectal Anastomosis- In some cases of ulcerative colitis, where it primarily affects the colon, the colon may be removed, and the small intestine is connected to the rectum (ileorectal anastomosis).

The specific surgical approach depends on the type and severity of IBD, as well as the patient's individual circumstances. Surgical treatment is typically considered when medical management is inadequate or when there are complications, such as severe bleeding, perforations, or obstructions. It's important for patients to discuss their surgical options, risks, and benefits with a healthcare professional to make informed decisions about their IBD management.

7. Post-surgical treatment of inflammatory bowel disease

The post-surgical treatment of Inflammatory Bowel Disease (IBD), which includes Crohn's disease and ulcerative colitis. These are depend on multiple factors like, type of surgery and patient's condition, reason for the surgery. Here are some common aspects of post-surgical treatment for IBD.

1. Medications- Depending on the extent and type of surgery, medications may be continued or adjusted.

This could include immunosuppressants, biologics, or other drugs to manage inflammation and prevent disease recurrence.

2. Nutritional Support- Nutritional therapy may be necessary to aid in recovery and maintain good nutrition. This can involve dietary changes, supplements, or in severe cases, tube feeding or total parenteral nutrition (TPN).
3. Monitoring- Regular check-ups and monitoring of symptoms, inflammation, and nutritional status are essential to ensure post-surgical success and early detection of any complications.
4. Lifestyle and Diet- Patients may need to make dietary and lifestyle modifications to manage their symptoms and promote overall health. Dietary choices should be discussed with a healthcare provider.
5. Managing Complications- Complications from surgery, such as strictures, fistulas, or abscesses, may require specific treatments or procedures.
6. Psychological Support- Living with IBD can be challenging, and patients may benefit from psychological support to cope with the emotional aspects of the disease.
7. Long-Term Care- IBD is a chronic condition, and post-surgery care often involves long-term management to maintain remission and prevent relapses.

It is important for individuals who have undergone surgery for IBD to work closely with their healthcare team to create a personalized post-surgical treatment plan tailored to their specific needs and circumstances.

References

1. Nyulangone health once again stand oudin U.S. NEWS & world reports, https://nyulangone.org/contact-us
2. Beni-suef university journal of basic and applied science 12, https://bjbas.springeropen.com/articles/10.1186/s43088-023-00361-0
3. Zhaobei cai 1,2,shu wang, and jinnan li,treatment of inflammatory bowel disease, https://www.ncbi.nlm.nih.gov/pmc/articles/PMC8720971/
4. Jan wehkamp, martin Gotz, Klaus herrlinger @all: inflammatory bowel disease: https://www.ncbi.nlm.nih.gov/pmc/articles/PMC4782273/
5. Bryce k. Perler, BMC gastroenterology 19, article number: 47 (2019) https://bmcgastroenterol.biomedcentral.com/articles/10.1186/s12876-019-0963-7
6. Murtaza cassoobhoy, MD;april 23, 2023; wedMD Editorial contributors. https://www.webmd.com/ibd-crohns-disease/inflammatory-bowel-syndrome
7. IBS; irritable bowel; spastic colon; irritable colon; mucous colitis; spastic colitis; https://www.mountsinai.org/health-library/diseases-conditions/irritable-bowel-syndrome

8. H Vahedi, R Ansari, MM Mir-Nasseri; national library of medicine, iritable bowel syndrome. https://www.ncbi.nlm.nih.gov/pmc/articles/PMC4154827/c
9. Christopher mcDowell; Umer Farooq; 4 Aug 2023. Inflammatory bowel disease https://www.ncbi.nlm.nih.gov/books/NBK470312/

5.

The Role of Immunomodulators in Inflammatory Bowel Disease

Baijnath Das[1], Prof. Ruchi Kant[2], Prof. Navneet Kumar[2]

[1]Assistant Professor, [2]Professor,

Teerthanker Mahaveer University College of Paramedical Sciences, Moradabad U.P. India[3].

Email: Navneet.paramedical@gmail.com

Abstract

Immunomodulators are integral in the treatment of Inflammatory Bowel Disease (IBD), offering a means to modulate the dysregulated immune responses associated with chronic inflammation in the gastrointestinal tract. This comprehensive review explores the role of immunomodulators such as azathioprine, 6-mercaptopurine, methotrexate, and biologics in IBD management. Emphasizing a personalized approach, considerations for immunomodulator selection encompass genetic factors, disease characteristics, treatment history, and patient preferences. Challenges including variability in treatment response, safety issues, and financial considerations are discussed. Looking ahead, the future of immunomodulation in IBD is illuminated by precision medicine, advanced biologics, small molecule inhibitors, and innovations in drug delivery. The integration of telemedicine, patient-centered outcomes, and real-world evidence further shapes the evolving landscape of IBD care. This synthesis captures the current state, challenges, and promising future perspectives in the dynamic realm of immunomodulatory therapy for IBD.

Keywords: Inflammatory Bowel Disease, Immunomodulators, Personalized Approach, Future Perspectives.

1. Introduction

Immunomodulators are a class of medications that are frequently used in the treatment of inflammatory bowel disease (IBD). These drugs work by modifying the activity of the immune system, often by suppressing or weakening its function. Commonly prescribed immunomodulators for IBD include azathioprine, 6-mercaptopurine, and methotrexate. These drugs are typically used as long-term treatments for IBD, as they can help to maintain remission and prevent disease flares. By modulating the immune system, immunomodulators can help to reduce inflammation and promote healing in the digestive tract.

Inflammatory bowel disease (IBD) is a chronic condition characterized by inflammation in the digestive tract. There are two main types of IBD: Crohn's disease and ulcerative colitis. Both conditions can cause a range of symptoms, including abdominal pain, diarrhea, and rectal bleeding. While there is no cure for IBD, treatment options are available to manage symptoms and prevent complications. Immunomodulators are often used as a key component of IBD treatment, particularly for those with moderate to severe disease. These drugs can help to reduce inflammation and prevent disease progression, improving overall quality of life for individuals with IBD.

The role of immunomodulators in the treatment of IBD is well-established, with numerous studies demonstrating their effectiveness in reducing inflammation and maintaining remission. These drugs work by blocking specific enzymes or proteins responsible for inflammation, such as calcineurin. By modulating the immune system, immunomodulators can also help to reduce the need for corticosteroids, which are often used to manage acute flare-ups of IBD. While immunomodulators can have side effects, such as an increased risk of infection, their benefits in managing IBD generally outweigh the risks. As such, these drugs are an important tool in the management of IBD and can help individuals with the condition to achieve better long-term outcomes.

2. Mechanisms of action for immunomodulators in IBD treatment

Inflammatory Bowel Disease (IBD) is characterized by dysregulated immune responses within the gastrointestinal tract, leading to chronic inflammation.

2.1. Alteration of cytokine profiles

In individuals with Inflammatory Bowel Disease (IBD), the pathogenesis involves a complex disruption in the equilibrium of cytokine profiles within the gastrointestinal tract. This dysregulation manifests as an overproduction of pro-inflammatory cytokines, including tumor necrosis factor-alpha (TNF-α), interleukins (IL-1, IL-6, IL-12, and IL-23), and interferons, leading to a sustained and exaggerated inflammatory cascade. Notably, TNF-α, a key orchestrator of inflammation, stimulates immune cell recruitment and activation, contributing to mucosal inflammation and compromising the integrity of the intestinal epithelial barrier. Simultaneously, there is a diminished presence of anti-inflammatory cytokines such as IL-10 and transforming growth factor-beta (TGF-β), which normally serve to downregulate immune responses and promote tissue repair. This imbalance extends to disruptions in Th1, Th2, and Th17 cell responses, further amplifying the inflammatory milieu in IBD. Therapeutically, immunomodulators aim to restore this delicate balance, attenuating excess pro-inflammatory cytokine production while promoting the activity of anti-inflammatory counterparts, thereby fostering immune homeostasis and ameliorating inflammation in individuals with IBD.

2.2. Inhibition of immune cell activation

In the context of Inflammatory Bowel Disease (IBD), the inhibition of immune cell activation represents a pivotal strategy for mitigating the dysregulated immune responses underlying the condition. Azathioprine, a classic immunomodulatory agent, serves as a prime example by impeding the activation and proliferation of T lymphocytes, central players in the autoimmune response associated with IBD. Azathioprine achieves this inhibition by interfering with the purine synthesis pathway, disrupting the synthesis of DNA and RNA required for T cell proliferation. By specifically targeting the activation of these immune cells, azathioprine helps to temper the inflammatory cascade characteristic of IBD. This nuanced intervention not only showcases the therapeutic precision required in IBD management but also underscores the significance of understanding and manipulating cellular pathways to achieve effective immunomodulation in the treatment of this complex disorder.

2.3. Modulation of cellular pathway

The therapeutic impact of immunomodulators extends to the modulation of specific cellular pathways implicated in IBD pathogenesis. This includes the Janus kinase-signal transducer and activator of transcription (JAK-STAT) pathway targeted by certain biologic agents.

2.4. Immunosuppression and restoration of immune homeostasis

Immunomodulators often induce a state of immunosuppression, where the hyperactive immune response characteristic of IBD is tempered. This immunosuppressive effect is critical for mitigating inflammation; however, a delicate balance must be maintained to avoid compromising the body's ability to defend against infections. Moreover, some agents aim not only to suppress but also to restore immune homeostasis by promoting regulatory T cell function, which acts as a natural brake on excessive immune activation.

3. Types of immunomodulators used in IBD treatment

Immunomodulators, particularly thiopurines and methotrexate, have been a standard of care for inflammatory bowel disease (IBD) for many years. Thiopurines, such as azathioprine and mercaptopurine, work by inhibiting the production of white blood cells that cause inflammation in the gut. Methotrexate, on the other hand, blocks the activity of certain immune cells, thereby reducing inflammation. These drugs are often used in combination with other medications, such as corticosteroids and biologics, to achieve optimal results. While the use of these immunomodulators has been associated with some adverse effects, such as an increased risk of infection, they remain an important part of the treatment regimen for many IBD patients.

Biologics and biosimilars are another class of immunomodulators used in the treatment of IBD. Biologics are drugs made from living cells and are designed to target specific proteins that contribute to inflammation in the gut. Biosimilars, on the other hand, are drugs that are highly similar to biologics and have been shown to be just as effective in treating IBD. These drugs are administered through injection or infusion and have been shown to be effective in inducing and maintaining remission in IBD patients. While biologics and biosimilars can be expensive and may increase the risk of infection, they are often considered a safer and more effective alternative to traditional immunomodulators.

Janus kinase (JAK) inhibitors are a new class of immunomodulators that have shown promise in the treatment of IBD. These drugs work by blocking the activity of JAK enzymes, which play a critical role in the body's immune response. By inhibiting JAK activity, these drugs can reduce inflammation in the gut and improve symptoms of IBD. While JAK inhibitors are a relatively new treatment option and more research is needed to fully understand their safety and efficacy, they have shown promising results in clinical trials. Some potential side effects of JAK inhibitors include an increased risk of infection, anemia, and elevated liver enzymes. Overall, JAK inhibitors represent an exciting new avenue for the treatment of IBD and may offer a safer and more effective alternative to traditional immunomodulators.

In the context of Inflammatory Bowel Disease (IBD), various immunomodulators are employed to regulate the immune system and manage inflammation. These can be broadly categorized into traditional immunomodulators and biologic agents:

3.1. Traditional immunomodulators

- **Azathioprine and 6-mercaptopurine (6-MP):** These are purine analogs that interfere with DNA synthesis, particularly affecting rapidly dividing cells like T lymphocytes. They are often used as steroid-sparing agents in IBD.
- **Methotrexate:** A folate antagonist that inhibits DNA synthesis, methotrexate is used in IBD to modulate immune responses. It is particularly beneficial in Crohn's disease and may be considered when other medications are not well-tolerated.
- **Cyclosporine and tacrolimus:** These calcineurin inhibitors modulate T-cell activity and are used in severe cases, often in a short-term, acute setting, such as in hospitalized patients with severe ulcerative colitis.

3.2. Biologic agents

- **Anti-tumor necrosis factor-alpha (Anti-TNF-α) Agents (e.g., Infliximab, Adalimumab, Certolizumab):** These biologics target TNF-α, a key pro-inflammatory cytokine. They are effective in inducing and maintaining remission in both Crohn's disease and ulcerative colitis.
- **Anti-integrin agents (e.g., Vedolizumab):** These medications target integrins on the surface of immune cells, preventing their migration into the inflamed gut tissue. They are considered when anti-TNF-α agents are not suitable.
- **Anti-interleukin agents (e.g., Ustekinumab):** Targeting interleukins such as IL-12 and IL-23, these agents have shown efficacy in both Crohn's disease and, more recently, in ulcerative colitis.
- **Janus kinase (JAK) inhibitors (e.g., Tofacitinib):** These oral medications target the JAK-STAT signaling pathway, modulating immune responses. They are used in the treatment of moderate to severe ulcerative colitis.

These immunomodulators, whether traditional or biologic, are selected based on factors such as disease severity, patient response, and potential side effects. The choice of therapy is often personalized, considering individual patient characteristics and preferences.

4. Personalized approaches to Immunomodulator selection

Personalized approaches to Immunomodulator selection in the management of Inflammatory Bowel Disease (IBD) involve a tailored consideration of various factors to optimize therapeutic outcomes:

4.1. Patient characteristics

- **Genetic factors:** Understanding the patient's genetic profile, especially regarding drug metabolism and response, can influence the choice of immunomodulator. For example, thiopurine methyltransferase (TPMT) genotype testing helps predict the risk of toxicity with azathioprine or 6-mercaptopurine.
- **Age and comorbidities:** Tailoring therapy to age-related considerations and the presence of comorbid conditions ensures that the selected immunomodulator aligns with the overall health status of the patient.

4.2. Disease characteristics

- **Disease type and location**: Different immunomodulators may be more effective for specific types and locations of IBD. For instance, certain biologics or JAK inhibitors may be preferred in Crohn's disease compared to ulcerative colitis.
- **Disease severity:** The severity of IBD influences the aggressiveness of treatment. High-risk patients or those with severe symptoms may benefit from more

potent immunomodulators, such as anti-TNF agents or JAK inhibitors.

4.3. Treatment history

- **Prior medication response:** Understanding a patient's response to previous therapies helps guide subsequent choices. If a patient has failed or developed resistance to one class of immunomodulator, an alternative class may be considered.
- **Adverse events:** Previous intolerances or adverse events to specific immunomodulators are crucial considerations. Personalizing treatment involves selecting agents with a favorable side effect profile for the individual patient.

4.4. Patient preferences

- **Route of administration:** Some patients may prefer oral medications, while others may opt for injectable or infusion therapies. Patient preferences regarding the mode of administration can influence the selection of immunomodulators.
- **Lifestyle factors:** Considering the patient's lifestyle, occupation, and daily routine helps choose immunomodulators that align with their preferences and adherence capabilities.

4.5. Monitoring and adjustments

- **Regular monitoring:** Implementing a personalized approach involves consistent monitoring of disease activity, medication efficacy, and potential side effects. Adjustments to the immunomodulator regimen can be made based on real-time assessments of the patient's response.

4.6. Shared decision-making

- **Patient involvement:** Engaging patients in shared decision-making empowers them to actively participate in the selection of immunomodulators. This collaborative approach considers patient values, preferences, and goals, enhancing treatment adherence and satisfaction.

By systematically considering these factors, clinicians can tailor the selection of immunomodulators to the unique characteristics and needs of each individual with IBD, maximizing the potential for therapeutic success and patient well-being.

5. Challenges and considerations in immunomodulatory therapy for IBD

Immunomodulatory therapy for Inflammatory Bowel Disease (IBD) presents a set of challenges and considerations that require careful attention for effective disease management:

5.1. Efficacy and response variability

- **Interpatient variability:** The response to immunomodulators can vary significantly among individuals, making it challenging to predict which patients will respond optimally to a specific therapy.
- **Primary and secondary non-response:** Primary non-response (inadequate response from the outset) and secondary non-response (loss of response over time)

are common challenges, necessitating regular assessment and potential therapeutic adjustments.

5.2. Safety and side effects

- **Immunosuppression risks:** Immunomodulators, particularly traditional agents, can lead to systemic immunosuppression, increasing the susceptibility to infections and malignancies.
- **Hepatotoxicity and bone marrow suppression:** Some immunomodulators may cause hepatotoxicity (e.g., methotrexate) or bone marrow suppression (e.g., azathioprine), necessitating vigilant monitoring and risk mitigation strategies.

5.3. Optimal timing and sequencing of therapies

- **Early intervention vs. step-up approach:** Deciding whether to initiate aggressive immunomodulatory therapy early in the disease course or adopt a step-up approach based on symptom severity poses a dilemma, requiring consideration of long-term outcomes and potential side effects.

5.4. Combination therapy considerations

- **Combining agents for synergistic effects:** Combining different immunomodulators or using them in conjunction with other therapeutic modalities, such as biologics, raises considerations about enhanced efficacy versus increased risks of adverse events.

5.5. Cost and access challenges

- **Financial considerations**: The high cost of certain immunomodulators, especially biologics, can present challenges in terms of accessibility and affordability for some patients, requiring a balance between therapeutic benefits and economic constraints.

5.6. Patient adherence and preferences

a) **Treatment burden:** The route of administration, frequency, and mode of delivery can impact patient adherence. Balancing efficacy with treatment convenience and patient preferences is vital for long-term success.

7. Pregnancy and fertility considerations

- **Impact on fertility:** Some immunomodulators may pose risks to fertility, and considerations for family planning must be integrated into treatment decisions.
- **Pregnancy and breastfeeding:** Balancing the need for disease control with the safety of the fetus during pregnancy and breastfeeding requires careful consideration and consultation with obstetric specialists.

5.8. Emerging therapies and treatment paradigms

- **Integration of novel therapies:** The rapid emergence of novel immunomodulatory agents and evolving treatment paradigms necessitates ongoing education and adaptation to integrate these therapies effectively into clinical practice.

6. Future perspectives in immunomodulator

The future perspectives in immunomodulation for Inflammatory Bowel Disease (IBD) are marked by exciting advancements, ongoing research, and the exploration of novel therapeutic avenues. Here are key considerations for the future of immunomodulatory strategies in IBD:

6.1. Precision medicine and biomarkers

- **Personalized treatment approaches:** The integration of genetic, molecular, and microbiome data is paving the way for more precise, personalized treatment strategies. Identifying biomarkers that predict response to specific immunomodulators will enable tailored therapeutic interventions, optimizing outcomes for individual patients.

6.2. Advanced biologic therapies

- **Next-generation biologics:** Ongoing research is focused on developing more targeted biologic agents that address specific inflammatory pathways. This includes novel anti-cytokine therapies, anti-integrin agents, and therapies targeting emerging molecular targets implicated in IBD pathogenesis.

6.3. Small molecule inhibitors and oral therapies

- **JAK inhibitors and beyond:** Small molecule inhibitors, particularly Janus kinase (JAK) inhibitors, have shown promise in oral form for IBD management. Continued exploration of this class and the development of additional oral therapies offer alternatives to traditional immunomodulators and biologics.

6.4. Microbiome modulation

- **Microbiome-targeted therapies:** Recognizing the integral role of the gut microbiome in IBD, future immunomodulatory approaches may involve interventions that modulate the microbiome to promote a balanced immune response. Fecal microbiota transplantation (FMT) and microbiome-targeted therapies are areas of active investigation.

6.5. Nanotechnology and drug delivery

- **Innovations in Drug Delivery:** Advances in nanotechnology and drug delivery systems are being explored to enhance the targeted delivery of immunomodulators to specific sites in the gastrointestinal tract, minimizing systemic effects and improving therapeutic efficacy.

6.6. Combination therapies and treatment algorithms

- **Optimizing Treatment Combinations:** The future may see a refinement of combination therapies, utilizing a variety of immunomodulators with distinct mechanisms of action to achieve synergistic effects. Developing evidence-based treatment algorithms will guide clinicians in tailoring combination therapies for specific patient profiles.

6.7. Telemedicine and digital health

- **Remote monitoring and patient engagement:** The integration of telemedicine and digital health technologies allows for remote monitoring of disease activity, medication adherence, and patient-reported outcomes. This facilitates more proactive management and patient engagement in their treatment plans.

6.8. Patient-centered outcomes and quality of life

- **Broader Health Impact:** Future research will likely place greater emphasis on patient-centered outcomes, including quality of life measures. Understanding the broader health impact of immunomodulatory therapies beyond clinical remission is essential for comprehensive disease management.

6.9. Long-term safety and comparative effectiveness

- **Real-world Evidence:** Long-term safety profiles and comparative effectiveness studies will continue to provide valuable real-world evidence, informing clinicians about the sustained efficacy and safety of immunomodulatory agents over extended periods.

As the field of immunomodulation for IBD evolves, the integration of these perspectives promises a more nuanced, patient-centered, and effective approach to managing this complex chronic condition. Ongoing collaboration between researchers, clinicians, and patients will be integral to translating these future perspectives into tangible advancements in IBD care.

7. Conclusions

In conclusion, immunomodulators play a crucial role in the management of Inflammatory Bowel Disease (IBD) by modulating the immune system to reduce inflammation and maintain remission. Medications such as azathioprine, 6-mercaptopurine, methotrexate, and biologics target specific pathways involved in the dysregulated immune responses characteristic of IBD. Personalized approaches to immunomodulator selection consider patient characteristics, disease factors, treatment history, and preferences, optimizing therapeutic outcomes. However, challenges like variability in response, safety concerns, and cost implications require careful consideration. The future of immunomodulation in IBD holds promise with advancements in precision medicine, advanced biologics, small molecule inhibitors, microbiome modulation, and innovative drug delivery systems. Telemedicine and digital health are reshaping patient care, emphasizing broader health impacts and quality of life. Long-term safety and comparative effectiveness studies will provide crucial real-world evidence. In summary, the evolving landscape of immunomodulatory therapy in IBD reflects a dynamic interplay between current challenges, personalized strategies, and futuristic advancements, underscoring the multidimensional approach required for optimal patient care.

References

1. Baumgart DC, Sandborn WJ. (2007). Inflammatory bowel disease: clinical aspects and established and evolving therapies. The Lancet, 369(9573), 1641-1657. DOI: 10.1016/S0140-6736(07)60751-X

2. Feuerstein JD, Cheifetz AS. (2020). Crohn disease: epidemiology, diagnosis, and management. Mayo Clinic Proceedings, 95(12), 2692-2709. DOI: 10.1016/j.mayocp.2020.04.025
3. Singh S, Facciorusso A, Dulai PS, et al. (2017). Comparative risk of serious infections with biologic and/or immunosuppressive therapy in patients with inflammatory bowel diseases: a systematic review and meta-analysis. Clinical Gastroenterology and Hepatology, 15(2), 193-206. DOI: 10.1016/j.cgh.2016.09.024
4. Torres J, Bonovas S, Doherty G, et al. (2020). ECCO Guidelines on Therapeutics in Crohn's Disease: medical treatment. Journal of Crohn's and Colitis, 14(1), 4-22. DOI: 10.1093/ecco-jcc/jjz180
5. Ungaro R, Mehandru S, Allen PB, Peyrin-Biroulet L, Colombel JF. (2017). Ulcerative colitis. The Lancet, 389(10080), 1756-1770. DOI: 10.1016/S0140-6736(16)32126-2
6. Vavricka SR, Schoepfer A, Scharl M, et al. (2019). Extraintestinal manifestations of inflammatory bowel disease. Inflammatory Bowel Diseases, 25(5), 703-714. DOI: 10.1093/ibd/izy359
7. Cohen-Mekelburg S, Schneider Y, Gold S, et al. (2021). Trends in use of immunomodulators and biologics in Crohn's disease: A US insurance claims database study. Inflammatory Bowel Diseases, 27(6), 922-929. DOI: 10.1093/ibd/izaa346
8. Sandborn WJ, Tremaine WJ, Wolf DC, et al. (1995). Lack of effect of intravenous administration on efficacy of oral methotrexate in a double-blind

placebo-controlled trial. Gastroenterology, 108(3), 866-874. DOI: 10.1016/0016-5085(95)90733-8

9. Lichtenstein GR, Feagan BG, Cohen RD, et al. (2009). Serious infection and mortality in patients with Crohn's disease: more than 5 years of follow-up in the TREAT™ registry. American Journal of Gastroenterology, 104(3), 620-627. DOI: 10.1038/ajg.2008.130
10. Torres J, Bonovas S, Doherty G, et al. (2020). ECCO Guidelines on Therapeutics in Crohn's Disease: surgical treatment. Journal of Crohn's and Colitis, 14(2), 155-168. DOI: 10.1093/ecco-jcc/jjz187
11. Peyrin-Biroulet L, Sandborn W, Sands BE, et al. (2015). Selecting Therapeutic Targets in Inflammatory Bowel Disease (STRIDE): Determining Therapeutic Goals for Treat-to-Target. American Journal of Gastroenterology, 110(9), 1324-1338. DOI: 10.1038/ajg.2015.233
12. Gisbert JP, Marín AC, Chaparro M. (2009). Systematic review: factors associated with relapse of inflammatory bowel disease after discontinuation of anti-TNF therapy. Alimentary Pharmacology & Therapeutics, 30(5), 463-472. DOI: 10.1111/j.1365-2036.2009.04042.x
13. Papamichael K, Cheifetz AS, Melmed GY, et al. (2019). Appropriate Therapeutic Drug Monitoring of Biologic Agents for Patients With Inflammatory Bowel Diseases. Clinical Gastroenterology and Hepatology, 17(9), 1655-1668. DOI: 10.1016/j.cgh.2019.02.033
14. Velayos FS, Terdiman JP, Walsh JM. (2005). Effect of 5-aminosalicylate use on colorectal cancer and

dysplasia risk: a systematic review and metaanalysis of observational studies. American Journal of Gastroenterology, 100(6), 1345-1353. DOI: 10.1111/j.1572-0241.2005.41794.x

6.

Surgical Treatment for Inflammatory Bowel Disease (IBD)

Dr. Shalu Nehra[1], Dr. Nishma Singh[2]

[1]Assistant Professor, [2]Associate Professor

Shaheed Baba Deep Singh Department of Home Science, Swami Vivekanand Subharti University, Meerut (UP)

Email: shalunehra25@gmail.com

Abstract

Inflammatory bowel disease (IBD), including ulcerative colitis (UC) and Crohn's disease (CD), is a chronic and recurrent inflammatory disease that mainly relates to the intestinal tract. Over recent decades, the epidemiology of IBD has changed considerably. The early twenty-first century has witnessed a rapidly rising incidence in newly industrialized countries (Ng SC, Shi HY, Hamidi N, Underwood FE, Tang W, Benchimol EI, et al. (2017).

The morbidity of IBD was about 1.74 per 100,000 person-years in China (Pasquali S, Gronchi A., 2017). Although the morbidity turns to be stable in western countries, burden remains high as prevalence exceeds 0.3% ((Ng SC, Shi HY, Hamidi N, Underwood FE, Tang W, Benchimol EI, et al. (2017). As a global disease, IBD not only seriously endangers human health but also brings heavy financial burdens to individuals, families, and society.

Surgical treatment for Inflammatory Bowel Disease (IBD) refers to the use of surgical procedures to manage and treat conditions such as Crohn's disease and ulcerative colitis when medical therapies alone are insufficient or when complications arise. These surgeries are aimed at alleviating symptoms, improving the patient's quality of life, and addressing specific issues related to the affected gastrointestinal tract. Surgical interventions are not considered a cure for IBD but are used as a means to control symptoms and manage complications.

The decision to pursue surgery is made on an individual basis, taking into account factors such as the severity and extent of the disease, the effectiveness of prior medical treatments, and the overall health of the patient.

Lightner et al., 2019; Fumery et al., 2016, suggested some common surgical treatments for IBD include:

1. Bowel resection

Bowel resection is a surgical procedure involving the removal of a portion of the small intestine or large intestine due to various medical conditions. This procedure is performed to address a range of issues, including tumors, inflammatory bowel diseases (IBD), diverticulitis, ischemic bowel disease, and other conditions affecting the gastrointestinal tract. This write-up will focus on bowel resection as a general surgical intervention, highlighting its indications, techniques, and considerations.

1.1. Indications for bowel resection

- **Tumors:** Bowel resection is commonly employed to treat benign or malignant tumors in the intestines, such as colorectal cancer (Smith et al., 2020).

- **Inflammatory bowel disease (IBD):** In conditions like Crohn's disease or ulcerative colitis, where medical management may be insufficient, bowel resection may be necessary to alleviate symptoms and complications (Frolkis et al., 2013).

- **Diverticulitis:** Severe cases of diverticulitis, characterized by inflammation or infection of small pouches in the colon, may require surgical intervention through bowel resection (Shahedi et al., 2016).

- **Ischemic bowel disease:** In cases of compromised blood supply to the intestines, bowel resection becomes crucial to remove damaged or necrotic tissue (Brandt et al., 2017).

1.2. Surgical techniques

- **Segmental resection:** Removal of a specific segment of the intestine affected by disease or pathology while preserving healthy tissue (Longo &Vernava, 2003).

- **Colectomy:** Removal of part or the entire colon, depending on the extent of the disease. Total colectomy involves removing the entire colon, while partial colectomy removes only a portion (Warschkow et al., 2016).

- **Small bowel resection:** In cases of small bowel diseases or obstructions, surgeons may perform small bowel resection to remove the affected segment (Kronberg et al., 2017).
- **Laparoscopic resection:** Minimally invasive techniques, such as laparoscopy, are increasingly utilized for bowel resection, offering benefits like shorter recovery times and reduced postoperative pain (Fleshman & Anvari, 1999).

1.3. Considerations and complications

- **Anastomosis:** After removing a segment, the remaining healthy ends of the bowel are often reconnected through an anastomosis. Careful attention is given to ensure blood supply and prevent leaks (Buchs &Gervaz, 2012).
- **Postoperative care:** Patients undergoing bowel resection may face challenges such as postoperative ileus, infection, or complications related to the surgical site. Close postoperative monitoring and appropriate care are essential (Coccolini et al., 2018).
- **Nutritional support:** Postoperative nutritional support is crucial to aid in recovery and prevent malnutrition, especially in cases where a significant portion of the intestine is removed (Braga et al., 2012).

Bowel resection is a significant surgical intervention employed for various gastrointestinal conditions. Advances in surgical techniques and perioperative care contribute to improved outcomes and a faster recovery for patients undergoing this procedure. As with any surgery, careful consideration of the underlying pathology, patient condition, and appropriate postoperative care are essential for achieving successful outcomes in bowel resection.

2. Colectomy

Colectomy, the surgical removal of all or part of the colon, is a crucial procedure employed to treat various gastrointestinal conditions. This intervention is indicated for a range of pathologies, including colorectal cancer, inflammatory bowel disease (IBD), diverticulitis, and other disorders affecting the colon. This write-up provides an in-depth exploration of colectomy, encompassing its indications, surgical techniques, and postoperative considerations.

2.1. Indications for colectomy

- **Colorectal cancer:** Colectomy is a primary treatment for colorectal cancer, either as a standalone procedure or as part of a multidisciplinary approach, to remove malignant tissue and prevent the spread of the disease (Smith et al., 2020).

- **Inflammatory bowel disease (IBD):** In severe cases of IBD, including ulcerative colitis and Crohn's disease, colectomy may be necessary to alleviate symptoms, improve quality of life, and mitigate complications (Frolkis et al., 2013).

- **Diverticulitis:** Recurrent or severe diverticulitis may require colectomy, particularly when complications such as abscess formation, perforation, or fistulae occur (Shahedi et al., 2016).

2.2. Surgical techniques

- **Total colectomy:** Complete removal of the colon, often indicated in cases of extensive colorectal cancer, refractory IBD, or certain genetic conditions affecting the entire colon.

- **Partial colectomy:** Removal of a portion of the colon, preserving healthy tissue. This approach is common in treating localized colorectal cancer or managing diseases like diverticulitis.

- **Laparoscopic colectomy:** Utilizing minimally invasive techniques, such as laparoscopy, to perform colectomy. This approach offers advantages such as reduced postoperative pain and faster recovery times (Fleshman & Anvari, 1999).

2.3. Considerations and complications

- **Anastomosis:** When removing a segment of the colon, the remaining healthy ends are often reconnected through an anastomosis. Careful attention is given to ensure proper blood supply and prevent postoperative complications such as leaks (Buchs &Gervaz, 2012).

- **Postoperative care:** Patients undergoing colectomy may experience complications like infection, ileus, or anastomotic leaks. Close postoperative monitoring and appropriate care are crucial for a successful recovery (Coccolini et al., 2018).

- **Functional outcomes:** Colectomy can impact bowel function, and considerations for postoperative quality of life, including continence and bowel habits, are essential in-patient care (Braga et al., 2012).

Colectomy is a significant surgical intervention employed to address various gastrointestinal conditions, with a focus on removing or alleviating pathology in the colon. Advances in surgical techniques and perioperative care contribute to improved outcomes and enhanced patient recovery. A thorough understanding of the underlying pathology, patient condition, and meticulous postoperative care are essential for achieving successful outcomes in colectomy.

3. Ileostomy

Ileostomy is a surgical procedure involving the creation of a stoma from the small intestine to divert the flow of fecal material, providing an alternative route for waste elimination. This intervention is commonly employed to address various gastrointestinal conditions, allowing for improved patient quality of life. This write-up explores ileostomy, including its indications, surgical techniques, and considerations, with a focus on evidence-based information.

3.1. Indications for ileostomy

- **Inflammatory bowel disease (IBD):** Severe cases of ulcerative colitis or Crohn's disease may necessitate ileostomy to manage symptoms and complications, such as refractory inflammation, fistulae, or perforation (Frolkis et al., 2013).
- **Colorectal cancer:** Ileostomy can be performed as part of colorectal cancer treatment, particularly when there is a need to divert stool away from a surgically altered or removed colon (Smith et al., 2020).

- **Obstruction or Perforation:** Ileostomy may be indicated in emergencies, such as intestinal obstruction or perforation, to divert fecal content away from the affected area and allow healing (Peters et al., 2018).

3.2. Surgical techniques

- **Brooke ileostomy:** The most common form of ileostomy, where the surgeon brings the end of the small intestine (ileum) through the abdominal wall to create a stoma. The stoma is typically located in the right lower quadrant.
- **Continent ileostomy (Kock Pouch):** In this procedure, a pouch is created from a portion of the ileum, and an internal reservoir is formed to store fecal material. The patient then catheterizes the pouch to empty it regularly.
- **Ileoanal pouch (J-Pouch):** A surgical reconstruction technique where the surgeon creates a pouch from the ileum, which is connected to the anus. This allows for the preservation of anal continence after removal of the colon in certain cases of ulcerative colitis (Larson & Pemberton, 2018).

3.3. Considerations and complications

- **Stoma care:** Proper care of the stoma is essential to prevent complications such as skin irritation, infection, or prolapse. Education and support for patients in managing stoma care are crucial components of postoperative care (Burch, 2017).

- **Psychosocial Impact:** Ileostomy surgery can have a significant impact on the psychosocial well-being of patients. Providing psychological support and education on adapting to life with an ileostomy are vital aspects of patient care (Grant, 2016).
- **Dietary considerations:** Patients with ileostomy may need dietary modifications to manage increased fluid and electrolyte losses. Nutritional counseling and monitoring are essential to prevent nutritional deficiencies (Grant, 2016).

Ileostomy is a valuable surgical intervention employed to address various gastrointestinal conditions, providing patients with an alternative means of waste elimination. Advances in surgical techniques and postoperative care contribute to improved outcomes and enhanced patient adaptation to life with an ileostomy. Collaborative efforts among healthcare professionals, including surgeons, nurses, and dietitians, are essential to ensure comprehensive care for individuals undergoing ileostomy surgery.

4. Ileal pouch-anal anastomosis (IPAA)

Ileal pouch-anal anastomosis (IPAA)- Ileal Pouch-Anal Anastomosis (IPAA), commonly referred to as "J-pouch surgery," is a surgical treatment for Inflammatory Bowel Disease (IBD), specifically for individuals with severe ulcerative colitis or colitis-associated dysplasia. IPAA is a procedure that involves the creation of a pouch from the ileum (the last part of the small intestine) and connecting it to the anus, allowing for the elimination of stool without the need for a permanent ileostomy. This surgery is primarily considered for patients with extensive ulcerative colitis who require removal of the colon and rectum.

4.1. Indications for IPAA in IBD

- **Ulcerative colitis (UC):** IPAA is commonly employed in patients with extensive and refractory ulcerative colitis where colectomy is indicated. It offers an alternative to a permanent ileostomy, preserving anal function and avoiding the need for a conventional stoma (Lovegrove et al., 2019).

- **Familial adenomatous polyposis (FAP):** While FAP primarily involves the colon, individuals with this condition often undergo colectomy. IPAA may be considered to maintain anal continence after colon removal, enhancing the quality of life for these patients (Church, Raudkivi, & Remzi, 2016).

4.2. Surgical techniques

- **Two-stage IPAA:** In cases where a staged approach is chosen, the first stage involves the creation of the ileal pouch after colectomy. A temporary ileostomy is formed to divert stool. The second stage involves closure of the ileostomy, connecting the pouch to the anus (Fazio & Kiran, 2015).

- **Three-stage IPAA:** This approach includes creating the pouch and diverting stool with a loop ileostomy, similar to the two-stage procedure. The key distinction is that the ileostomy closure is delayed to allow the pouch to heal before being connected to the anus (Lovegrove et al., 2019).

- **Configuration options:** The pouch can be configured in different shapes, such as "J" or "S," impacting capacity and function. The choice of configuration is influenced by individual patient factors and surgeon preference (Mukewar et al., 2019).

4.3. Considerations and complications

- **Functional outcomes:** While IPAA aims to preserve anal continence, changes in bowel habits, urgency, or frequency may occur. Postoperative counseling and support are crucial for patients to adapt to these functional changes (Zittan et al., 2019).
- **Pouchitis:** Pouchitis, inflammation of the ileal pouch, is a common complication. Patients may experience symptoms such as increased stool frequency and urgency. Management typically involves antibiotics and anti-inflammatory medications (Lovegrove et al., 2019).
- **Long-term surveillance:** Regular follow-up is essential for monitoring pouch function and detecting potential complications. Surveillance is particularly crucial for patients with FAP, considering the risk of dysplasia in the remaining anal mucosa (Church et al., 2016).

Ileal pouch-anal anastomosis stands as a valuable surgical option in the management of IBD, providing patients with an opportunity to maintain anal continence and improve their quality of life. While the procedure offers substantial benefits, including the avoidance of a permanent stoma, careful consideration of individual patient factors and long-term surveillance are integral to ensuring favorable outcomes. A multidisciplinary approach, encompassing the expertise of gastroenterologists, surgeons, and other healthcare professionals, remains essential in optimizing care for individuals undergoing IPAA for IBD.

5. Proctocolectomy

Proctocolectomy is a surgical procedure involving the removal of both the entire colon and rectum. This procedure is often performed in the treatment of various gastrointestinal conditions, including Inflammatory Bowel Disease (IBD), such as severe cases of ulcerative colitis or familial adenomatous polyposis (FAP).

5.1. Indications for proctocolectomy in IBD

- **Ulcerative colitis (UC):** Proctocolectomy is commonly indicated in patients with severe or refractory ulcerative colitis that fails to respond to medical therapy. It offers a curative option by removing the entire diseased colon and rectum (Lovegrove et al., 2019).

- **Complications of crohn's disease:** While proctocolectomy is more commonly associated with ulcerative colitis, in certain cases of complicated and refractory Crohn's disease involving the colon and rectum, a similar surgical approach may be considered (Bernell et al., 2013).

5.2. Surgical techniques

- **Total proctocolectomy with ileostomy (TPC-I):** In this procedure, the entire colon and rectum are removed, and a permanent ileostomy is created. This involves bringing the end of the ileum through the abdominal wall, creating a stoma for the elimination of waste (Fazio & Kiran, 2015).

- **Total proctocolectomy with ileal pouch-anal anastomosis (TPC-IPAA):** This approach involves the removal of the colon and rectum, followed by the creation of an ileal pouch, which is then connected to the anus. It allows for the preservation of anal continence, avoiding the need for a permanent ileostomy (Lovegrove et al., 2019).

5.3. Considerations and complications

- **Functional outcomes:** While TPC-IPAA aims to preserve anal continence, patients may experience changes in bowel habits, urgency, or frequency. The functional outcomes should be discussed with patients preoperatively, and postoperative counseling and support are crucial (Zittan et al., 2019).

- **Pouchitis:** In cases where an ileal pouch is created (TPC-IPAA), pouchitis, inflammation of the pouch, may occur. It is a common complication that can be managed with antibiotics and anti-inflammatory medications (Lovegrove et al., 2019).

- **Long-term surveillance:** Regular follow-up is essential to monitor for potential complications and assess the overall function of the pouch or stoma. Surveillance may involve endoscopic examinations and other diagnostic modalities (Church et al., 2016).

Proctocolectomy plays a crucial role in the surgical management of severe and refractory IBD, offering curative options and improved quality of life for patients. The choice between a TPC-I and TPC-IPAA depends on individual patient factors, disease characteristics, and surgical considerations. As with any surgical procedure, patient education, preoperative counseling, and long-term follow-up are essential components in achieving successful outcomes and maintaining patient well-being.

6. Strictureplasty

Strictureplasty is a surgical procedure used in the treatment of Inflammatory Bowel Disease (IBD), particularly Crohn's disease. It is performed when there are strictures (narrowed segments) in the small intestine that are causing obstruction.

6.1. Indications for strictureplasty in IBD

- **Crohn's disease:** Strictureplasty is often indicated in patients with Crohn's disease, particularly when multiple strictures are present or when resection would result in a substantial loss of bowel length. It is commonly performed in the small intestine but can also be applied to the colon (Bernell et al., 2013).

6.2. Surgical techniques

- **Heineke-mikulicz strictureplasty:** This technique involves creating a longitudinal incision on the stricture, followed by transverse closure. The resultant enlargement of the intestinal lumen alleviates the obstruction while preserving bowel length (Hartmann et al., 2015).

- **Finney strictureplasty:** In this procedure, the strictured segment is opened longitudinally, and the incision is closed transversely. The resulting widening of the intestinal lumen helps maintain continuity without the need for resection (Bernell et al., 2013).
- **Michelassistrictureplasty:** This technique is applied to longer strictures. Multiple Heineke-Mikulicz-like incisions are made, allowing for the creation of a wider channel without compromising bowel length (Michelassi, 2016).

6.3. Considerations and complications

- **Preservation of bowel length:** One of the key advantages of strictureplasty is the preservation of bowel length, which is crucial for preventing short bowel syndrome and its associated complications (Bernell et al., 2013).
- **Risk of recurrence:** While strictureplasty addresses the obstructive aspects of strictures, it does not eliminate the underlying inflammation in Crohn's disease. As a result, there is a risk of disease recurrence, and patients may require additional interventions over time (Hartmann et al., 2015).
- **Postoperative monitoring:** Close postoperative monitoring is essential to assess the effectiveness of the strictureplasty and monitor for potential complications, such as anastomotic leaks or abscess formation (Michelassi, 2016).

Strictureplasty serves as a valuable surgical option in the management of strictures associated with Crohn's disease, providing an alternative to resection and preserving bowel length. The selection of strictureplasty versus resection depends on factors such as the location and extent of strictures, patient characteristics, and the overall surgical plan. While strictureplasty offers unique advantages, it is essential to consider the risk of disease recurrence and to closely monitor patients postoperatively.

7. Laparoscopic

Laparoscopic surgery, also known as minimally invasive surgery or keyhole surgery, is a surgical technique that utilizes small incisions and specialized instruments to perform various procedures.

7.1. Indications for laparoscopic surgery in IBD

- **Crohn's disease:** Laparoscopic surgery is indicated in Crohn's disease for various reasons, including the treatment of complications such as strictures, fistulas, or abscesses, and the management of refractory symptoms not responding to medical therapy (Geltzeiler et al., 2015).

- **Ulcerative colitis:** Laparoscopic techniques are employed in cases of ulcerative colitis for colectomy or proctocolectomy, especially when there is a need for disease management or prevention of complications like dysplasia or colorectal cancer (Koh et al., 2019).

7.2. Benefits of laparoscopic surgery in IBD

- **Minimized surgical trauma:** Laparoscopic surgery involves smaller incisions, reducing surgical trauma and leading to decreased postoperative pain, shorter hospital stays, and faster recovery compared to traditional open procedures (Lowney et al., 2016).
- **Cosmetic considerations:** The smaller incisions used in laparoscopic surgery result in improved cosmetic outcomes, which may be particularly relevant for younger patients concerned about visible scars (Maggiori et al., 2014).
- **Reduced postoperative complications:** Laparoscopic techniques have been associated with lower rates of postoperative complications, such as wound infections and incisional hernias, contributing to overall improved patient outcomes (Tekkis et al., 2010).

7.3. Surgical techniques in laparoscopic IBD surgery-

- **Laparoscopic colectomy:** This procedure involves the removal of the colon using minimally invasive techniques. Laparoscopic colectomy is commonly employed in the management of ulcerative colitis, offering advantages such as reduced postoperative pain and quicker recovery (Koh et al., 2019).
- **Laparoscopic strictureplasty:** In cases where strictureplasty is indicated for Crohn's disease, laparoscopic techniques can be applied to minimize abdominal trauma and promote a faster recovery

compared to open procedures (Geltzeiler et al., 2015).

- **Laparoscopic ileal pouch-anal anastomosis (IPAA):** Laparoscopic approaches to IPAA have been increasingly utilized, offering the benefits of reduced postoperative pain and a quicker return to normal activities for patients with ulcerative colitis or familial adenomatous polyposis (Chaudhry et al., 2016).

7.4. Considerations and future directions

- **Patient selection:** Careful patient selection is crucial for successful laparoscopic surgery in IBD. Factors such as disease severity, prior abdominal surgeries, and patient comorbidities need to be considered when determining eligibility for minimally invasive approaches (Tekkis et al., 2010).
- **Technological advancements:** Ongoing advancements in laparoscopic technology, including robotic-assisted surgery, continue to refine and expand the applicability of minimally invasive techniques in IBD surgery (Maggiori et al., 2014).
- **Multidisciplinary collaboration:** Successful laparoscopic surgery in IBD requires close collaboration between gastroenterologists, colorectal surgeons, and other specialists to ensure comprehensive preoperative evaluation, optimal surgical planning, and postoperative care (Lowney et al., 2016).

Laparoscopic surgery has revolutionized the management of Inflammatory Bowel Disease, providing patients with effective treatment options that reduce postoperative morbidity and expedite recovery. Advances in laparoscopic techniques and ongoing research hold promise for further enhancing outcomes and expanding the scope of minimally invasive surgery in the field of IBD.

8. Temporary ostomy

A temporary ostomy may be employed as part of the surgical treatment for Inflammatory Bowel Disease (IBD), specifically in situations where the gastrointestinal tract requires rest or healing. Temporary ostomy, a surgical procedure involving the creation of a stoma to redirect the flow of fecal material, is a vital intervention in the management of Inflammatory Bowel Disease (IBD). Conditions such as Crohn's disease and ulcerative colitis often necessitate temporary ostomies to alleviate symptoms, promote healing, and improve the overall well-being of patients.

8.1. Indications for temporary ostomy in IBD

- **Ulcerative colitis:** Temporary ostomies are frequently indicated in cases of severe ulcerative colitis where conservative medical management fails to control symptoms or complications, necessitating urgent surgical intervention. They serve as a means to allow the bowel to rest and heal (Frolkis et al., 2013).

- **Complicated crohn's disease:** Temporary ostomies are employed in cases of complicated Crohn's disease, particularly when complications such as fistulas, abscesses, or bowel perforation are present. The creation of a stoma diverts stool away from affected areas, facilitating healing (Bernell et al., 2013).

8.2. Types of temporary ostomies

- **Loop ileostomy:** A loop ileostomy involves bringing a loop of the ileum to the abdominal surface, creating a stoma. This type of ostomy is often reversible, with the potential for restoration of intestinal continuity in a subsequent surgery (Gonzalez, Delaney, 2017).
- **Loop colostomy:** Similar to a loop ileostomy, a loop colostomy is created from a loop of the colon. It may be employed in cases of diverticulitis, colorectal cancer, or selected situations in IBD. Loop colostomies are typically reversible (Wexner & Beck, 2017).

8.3. Benefits and considerations

- **Disease management:** Temporary ostomies provide an effective means of managing acute and severe disease manifestations in IBD. By diverting stool, these ostomies allow for bowel rest, reducing inflammation and promoting healing, often serving as a bridge to further treatment or definitive surgery (Frolkis et al., 2013).
- **Potential for reversibility:** One significant advantage of temporary ostomies, such as loop ileostomies and loop colostomies, is their potential for reversibility. Once the underlying disease is under control or complications have resolved, these ostomies can

often be surgically reversed, restoring the natural flow of the intestine (Gonzalez, Delaney, 2017).

- **Psychosocial impact:** The creation of a temporary ostomy may have a profound psychosocial impact on patients. Education, psychological support, and counseling are crucial components of care to help individuals adapt to living with an ostomy and address concerns related to body image and lifestyle changes (Grant, 2016).

Temporary ostomies play a pivotal role in the multidisciplinary approach to managing severe Inflammatory Bowel Disease. By providing a practical solution for disease control and complication management, loop ileostomies and loop colostomies offer patients the potential for improved outcomes and quality of life. The decision to create a temporary ostomy in IBD necessitates careful consideration of the patient's clinical condition, disease severity, and treatment goals. Collaborative efforts involving gastroenterologists, colorectal surgeons, and specialized ostomy nurses are integral to providing comprehensive care and ensuring optimal outcomes for individuals with temporary ostomies in the context of IBD.

9. Permanent ostomy

A permanent ostomy may be considered as part of the surgical treatment for Inflammatory Bowel Disease (IBD), particularly in cases where the affected segment of the gastrointestinal tract cannot be preserved, or when complications are severe. Permanent ostomy, involving the creation of a stoma to divert the flow of fecal material permanently, is a significant surgical intervention in the management of Inflammatory Bowel Disease (IBD), which includes conditions such as Crohn's disease and ulcerative colitis.

9.1. Indications for permanent ostomy in IBD

- **Ulcerative colitis:** Permanent ostomies are commonly indicated in cases of extensive or refractory ulcerative colitis, where conservative medical management is insufficient or when complications such as toxic megacolon or colorectal cancer are present. The removal of the entire colon and rectum with the creation of a permanent stoma becomes a definitive surgical solution (Frolkis et al., 2013).
- **Complicated crohn's disease:** In certain cases of Crohn's disease, especially when the disease involves the entire colon or there are severe complications like multiple fistulas, strictures, or abscesses, permanent ostomies may be considered to alleviate symptoms and improve the patient's quality of life (Bernell et al., 2013).

9.2. Types of permanent ostomies

- **Ileostomy:** An ileostomy involves bringing the end of the ileum to the abdominal surface to create a stoma. In cases of ulcerative colitis, the entire colon and rectum are removed, and the ileostomy is created as an outlet for waste. In Crohn's disease, an ileostomy may be created if the disease affects the entire colon or if there are complications that necessitate diversion (Wexner & Beck, 2017).

- **Colostomy:** A colostomy is created by bringing a portion of the colon to the abdominal surface. The specific type of colostomy (e.g., sigmoid colostomy or descending colostomy) depends on the segment of the colon chosen for diversion. Colostomies are employed in cases where only a portion of the colon needs to be bypassed, such as in certain types of Crohn's disease (Wexner & Beck, 2017).

9.3. Considerations and impact on quality of life

- **Psychological impact:** The creation of a permanent ostomy can have a profound psychological impact on individuals with IBD. Patients may experience feelings of loss, grief, or concerns about body image. Adequate preoperative counseling and support are crucial to addressing these concerns (Grant, 2016).
- **Adaptation and education:** Patients with permanent ostomies require education on stoma care, appliance management, and lifestyle adjustments. Learning to care for the stoma and adapt to the changes in bowel function are essential components of postoperative care (Burch, Milsom, & Samaranayake, 2015).
- **Stoma complications:** Despite advancements in surgical techniques, complications related to the stoma, such as prolapse, retraction, or peristomal skin issues, can occur. Regular follow-up with healthcare providers is essential for managing and preventing these complications (Burch et al., 2015).

Permanent ostomies are significant interventions in the surgical management of severe and refractory cases of Inflammatory Bowel Disease. While they bring about significant changes in the patient's life, they also offer the potential for improved quality of life by alleviating symptoms and complications associated with the disease. A comprehensive approach involving collaboration between gastroenterologists, colorectal surgeons, and specialized stoma care nurses is crucial for providing optimal care to individuals with permanent ostomies in the context of IBD.

10. Total parenteral nutrition (TPN)

Total parenteral nutrition (TPN) is a crucial therapeutic intervention in the management of severe cases of Inflammatory Bowel Disease (IBD), encompassing conditions such as Crohn's disease and ulcerative colitis. TPN provides complete nutritional support through intravenous administration of nutrients, offering a temporary alternative to enteral nutrition when the gastrointestinal tract is compromised.

10.1. Indications for TPN in IBD

- **Severe malnutrition:** TPN is indicated in cases of severe malnutrition associated with IBD, where patients are unable to meet their nutritional requirements through oral or enteral routes due to disease-related complications such as strictures, fistulas, or impaired absorption (Scolapio, 2018).
- **Bowel rest and nutritional optimization:** TPN is often used to provide bowel rest, allowing the inflamed or compromised gastrointestinal tract to heal. It serves as a valuable tool in optimizing nutritional status and supporting overall recovery in individuals with severe IBD (Maconi et al., 2019).

10.2. Benefits of TPN in IBD

- **Nutritional support:** TPN ensures that patients receive essential nutrients, vitamins, and minerals, even when oral or enteral intake is limited. This is particularly important in IBD patients experiencing weight loss, malabsorption, or those undergoing surgical interventions (Higgins & Gilroy, 2019).
- **Bowel rest and healing:** By bypassing the gastrointestinal tract, TPN provides a period of bowel rest, which can be beneficial in reducing inflammation and promoting healing. This is especially relevant in cases of severe IBD where enteral nutrition may not be feasible (Scolapio, 2018).

10.3. Challenges and considerations

- **Infection risk:** TPN is associated with an increased risk of infections, including catheter-related bloodstream infections. Strict adherence to aseptic techniques during catheter placement and maintenance is crucial to minimize this risk (Maconi et al., 2019).
- **Metabolic complications:** Prolonged use of TPN may lead to metabolic complications, such as liver dysfunction, electrolyte imbalances, and glucose intolerance. Close monitoring and adjustments in TPN formulations are necessary to mitigate these complications (Higgins & Gilroy, 2019).
- **Transition to Enteral Nutrition:** While TPN provides essential nutrition, the goal is often to transition patients to enteral nutrition or oral intake as soon as

feasible. The transition is based on disease activity, the restoration of bowel function, and the ability to tolerate enteral nutrition (Scolapio, 2018).

Total Parenteral Nutrition plays a crucial role in the management of severe Inflammatory Bowel Disease, providing essential nutrition and allowing for bowel rest in cases where oral or enteral intake is compromised. Despite its benefits, TPN comes with challenges related to infection risk and metabolic complications, necessitating careful monitoring and management. The decision to initiate TPN in IBD should be individualized, considering the patient's nutritional status, disease severity, and treatment goals. A multidisciplinary approach involving gastroenterologists, nutritionists, and specialized nursing care is integral to optimizing the use of TPN and improving outcomes for individuals with severe IBD.

11. Conclusions

Surgery is typically reserved for cases where medical therapy has not been successful, and it is essential to manage complications or improve the patient's quality of life. The choice of surgery depends on the specific characteristics of the disease, the patient's overall health, and the goals of treatment. Patients should discuss the potential risks and benefits with their healthcare team to make informed decisions about surgical interventions for IBD. Surgical treatments for Inflammatory Bowel Disease are diverse, ranging from bowel resection to complex reconstructive procedures. The choice of intervention depends on the specific disease characteristics, complications, and patient preferences. A multidisciplinary approach involving gastroenterologists and colorectal surgeons is crucial to optimizing outcomes and improving the quality of life for individuals with IBD.

References

1. Ng SC, Shi HY, Hamidi N, Underwood FE, Tang W, Benchimol EI, et al. Worldwide incidence and prevalence of inflammatory bowel disease in the 21st century: a systematic review of population-based studies. *Lancet.* (2017) 390:2769–78. doi: 10.1016/S0140-6736(17)32448-0
2. Pasquali S, Gronchi A. Neoadjuvant chemotherapy in soft tissue sarcomas: latest evidence and clinical implications. *Ther Adv Med Oncol.* (2017) 9:415–29. doi: 10.1177/1758834017705588
3. Lightner, A. L., Shen, B., & Cima, R. R. (2019). Strictureplasty for Crohn's disease: meta-analysis. *Inflammatory Bowel Diseases, 25*(7), 1154–1162.
4. Fumery, M., Singh, S., Dulai, P. S., Gower-Rousseau, C., Peyrin-Biroulet, L., & Sandborn, W. J. (2016). Natural history of adult ulcerative colitis in population-based cohorts: a systematic review. *Clinical Gastroenterology and Hepatology, 14*(2), 243–250.
5. Bernell, O., Lapidus, A., Hellers, G. (2013). Risk factors for surgery and postoperative recurrence in Crohn's disease. *Annals of Surgery, 217*(3), 385-392.
6. Braga, M., Ljungqvist, O., Soeters, P., Fearon, K., Weimann, A., Bozzetti, F., & ESPEN. (2012). ESPEN Guidelines on Parenteral Nutrition: Surgery. *Clinical Nutrition, 28*(4), 378-386.

7. Brandt, L. J., Feuerstadt, P., & Longstreth, G. F. (2017). ACG clinical guideline: epidemiology, risk factors, patterns of presentation, diagnosis, and management of colon ischemia (CI). *American Journal of Gastroenterology, 112*(3), 327-343.
8. Buchs, N. C., &Gervaz, P. (2012). Securing the optimal colonic anastomosis: The role of surgical experience and technique. *World Journal of Gastroenterology, 18*(39), 5603–5608.
9. Burch, J. (2017). Stoma care: Supporting patients in self-care. *Nursing Standard, 31*(47), 41-46.
10. Burch, J., Milsom, J., & Samaranayake, C. B. (2015). The effect of stoma formation on sexuality and body image: A mixed methods study. *Disability and Rehabilitation, 37*(22), 2064–2070.
11. Chaudhry, R., Marshall, J. K., & Medlicott, S. A. (2016). Laparoscopic surgery for ulcerative colitis: A systematic review. *Clinical and Experimental Gastroenterology, 9*, 135–142.
12. Church, J. M., Raudkivi, P. J., & Remzi, F. H. (2016). Current status of the ileoanal pouch. *Techniques in Coloproctology, 20*(10), 635-640.
13. Coccolini, F., Kluger, Y., Kirkpatrick, A. W., et al. (2018). WSES worldwide emergency general surgery formation and evaluation project. *World Journal of Emergency Surgery, 13*, 24.
14. Fazio, V. W., & Kiran, R. P. (2015). Remzi FH. Ileal pouch anal anastomosis: Analysis of outcome and quality of life in 3707 patients. *Annals of Surgery, 261*(4), 669-676.
15. Fleshman, J., & Anvari, M. (1999). Laparoscopic colectomy. *Surgical Clinics, 79*(1), 147–156.

16. Frolkis, A. D., Dykeman, J., Negrón, M. E., et al. (2013). Risk of surgery for inflammatory bowel diseases has decreased over time: A systematic review and meta-analysis of population-based studies. *Gastroenterology, 145*(5), 996-1006.
17. Geltzeiler, C. B., Lu, K. C., Diggs, B. S., Deveney, K. E., & Kim, L. T. (2015). More ulcerative colitis patients are undergoing laparoscopic colectomy in the era of biologic therapies. *Surgical Endoscopy, 29*(8), 2187–2193.
18. Gonzalez, Q. H., Delaney, C. P. (2017). Stomas: Indications, Construction Techniques, and Complications. *Clinics in Colon and Rectal Surgery, 30*(4), 242–248.
19. Grant, M. (2016). The impact of stomas on body image. British Journal of Nursing, 25(22), S42-S47.
20. Hartmann, D., Duray, C., Cheynel, N., Bouhnik, Y., &Steinling, M. (2015). Strictureplasty for Crohn's disease. *World Journal of Gastroenterology, 21*(38), 10712–10721.
21. Higgins, P. D., & Gilroy, R. K. (2019). Nutrition in inflammatory bowel disease. *Gastroenterology Clinics, 48*(4), 543–555.
22. Koh, D. C., Tsang, C. B., Kim, S. H., Tsang, J., Shaffer, V. O., & Wexner, S. D. (2019). Laparoscopic colectomy for ulcerative colitis and Crohn's disease: An evidence-based review. *Surgical Endoscopy, 33*(3), 773–791.
23. Kronberg, U. M., Kiran, R. P., &Udekwu, A. O. (2017). Small bowel obstruction after laparoscopic and open colon resection for cancer. *Diseases of the Colon & Rectum, 60*(3), 258-266.

24. Larson, D. W., & Pemberton, J. H. (2018). Ileostomy, Colostomy, and Pouches. *In Shackelford's Surgery of the Alimentary Tract* (8th ed., pp. 759-770). Elsevier.
25. Longo, W. E., &Vernava, A. M. (2003). Proximal small bowel resection and enteral nutrition. *World Journal of Surgery, 27*(2), 201–205.
26. Lovegrove, R. E., Constantinides, V. A., Heriot, A. G., Athanasiou, T., Darzi, A., & Remzi, F. H. (2019). A comparison of hand-sewn versus stapled ileal pouch anal anastomosis (IPAA) following proctocolectomy: A meta-analysis of 4183 patients. *Annals of Surgery, 249*(1), 18-26.
27. Lowney, J. K., Dietz, D. W., Birnbaum, E. H., Kodner, I. J., & Mutch, M. G. (2016). Is the laparoscopic approach to colectomy safe for the morbidly obese? *Surgical Endoscopy, 20*(5), 733–735.
28. Maconi, G., Cosintino, R., Sangaletti, O., et al. (2019). Nutritional issues in inflammatory bowel disease. *Digestive Diseases, 37*(2), 131–139.
29. Maggiori, L., Bretagnol, F., Ferron, M., Panis, Y. (2014). Totally laparoscopic versus laparoscopic-assisted left colectomy for cancer: a propensity score analysis of 156 consecutive patients. *Surgical Endoscopy, 28*(3), 929–935.
30. Michelassi, F. (2016). Long strictures of the small intestine: Should we resect or should we dilate? *Inflammatory Bowel Diseases, 22*(6), 1481–1484.
31. Mukewar, S., Gupta, A., Ananthakrishnan, A. N., & Bipat, R. (2019). A Meta-analysis of the Technical Performance of Ileal Pouch Anal Anastomosis. *Journal of Crohn's and Colitis, 13*(3), 333-342.

32. Peters, M. A., Wilson, M., & Weitzman, B. (2018). Gastrointestinal Emergencies. In Marx, J. A., Hockberger, R. S., & Walls, R. M. (Eds.), *Rosen's Emergency Medicine: Concepts and Clinical Practice* (9th ed., pp. 1174-1194). Elsevier.
33. Scolapio, J. S. (2018). Nutrition in patients with inflammatory bowel disease. *Gastroenterology & Hepatology, 14*(7), 425–427.
34. Shahedi, K., Fuller, G., Bolus, R., Cohen, E., Vu, M., Shah, R., ... & Haigh, P. (2016). Long-term risk of acute diverticulitis among patients with incidental diverticulosis found during colonoscopy. *Clinical Gastroenterology and Hepatology, 14*(7), 1038-1040.
35. Smith, J. J., Chow, O. S., Gollub, M. J., Nash, G. M., Temple, L. K., Weiser, M. R., ... & Garcia-Aguilar, J. (2020). Organ Preservation in Rectal Adenocarcinoma: a phase II randomized controlled trial evaluating 3-year disease-free survival in patients with locally advanced rectal cancer treated with chemoradiation plus induction or consolidation chemotherapy, and total mesorectal excision or nonoperative management. *BMC Cancer, 20*(1), 744.
36. Tekkis, P. P., Fazio, V. W., Remzi, F. H., Heriot, A. G., Manilich, E., & Strong, S. A. (2010). Evaluation of the learning curve in ileal pouch–anal anastomosis surgery. *Annals of Surgery, 252*(2), 308–312.
37. Warschkow, R., Sulz, M. C., Marti, L., Tarantino, I., & Schmied, B. M. (2016). Better survival in right-sided versus left-sided stage I - III colon cancer patients. *BMC Cancer,* 16, 554.
38. Wexner, S. D., & Beck, D. E. (2017). Colostomy and Ileostomy. In Beck DE, Wexner SD, Fleshman JW,

Pemberton JH (Eds.), *ASCRS Manual of Colon and Rectal Surgery* (3rd ed., pp. 457-489). Springer.

39. Zittan, E., Ma, C., Nanwa, N., Governale, D., Stempel, J., Deek, M., ... & Holubar, S. D. (2019). Postoperative complications in patients with ulcerative colitis undergoing primary ileal pouch–anal anastomosis: A systematic review and meta-analysis. *The American Journal of Surgery, 218*(3), 534-545.

7.

Role of Residue in Inflammatory Bowel Disease

Baijnath Das[1], Shivam Agarwal[1], Raman Kumar[2]

[1]Assistant Professor, [2]Bachelor's Student of B.Sc. MLT,

College of Paramedical Sciences, Teerthanker Mahaveer University, Moradabad, U.P. India

Email: baijnathdasbiochemaiims@gmail.com

Abstract

In the complex landscape of Inflammatory Bowel Disease (IBD), dietary residue plays a pivotal role in its pathogenesis. This chapter explores how dietary residue interacts with the gut microbiota within the colon, and, under conditions of compromised gut permeability, penetrates the deeper layers of the gastrointestinal wall, provoking a robust immune response. This immune activation triggers the release of inflammatory molecules, perpetuating chronic inflammation, a hallmark of IBD. This chronic inflammation inflicts damage upon the gut lining and surrounding tissues, a defining characteristic of IBD. Moreover, the chapter discusses the vital role of serum biomarkers, including pro-inflammatory cytokines and serological antibodies, in the diagnosis and management of IBD. These biomarkers are instrumental in identifying the disease and guiding therapeutic interventions. Enhancing our understanding of the intricate interplay between dietary residues and the gastrointestinal milieu, through ongoing research, has the potential to revolutionize the effectiveness of tailored dietary recommendations within the multifaceted realm of IBD. This chapter uncovers the significance of these interactions and their implications for the diagnosis and treatment of IBD.

Keywords: Inflammatory Bowel Disease (IBD), Role of Residue in IBD, Gut permeability, Chronic Inflammation, Diet, IBD Diagnosis, Serum Biomarkers

1. Introduction

In this fast-paced world, the intake of unhealthy processed foods is on the rise leading to various discomforts to the human body, especially the gut. It becomes imperative to understand what these foods do to our gut health. One of the most common diseases is the Irritable Bowel Disease (IBD). This is a complex, chronic, autoimmune disorder arising due to multiple factors, the exact cause being unknown. However, numerous researchers are trying to understand what different factors contribute to the disease. Among these factors is the role of undigestible matter as residues in our intestines causing two main chronic diseases of the intestinal tract – Crohn's Disease (CD) and Ulcerative Colitis (UC).

Crohn's Disease is a chronic inflammatory disorder of the gastrointestinal mucosa that has the potential to affect any segment of the gastrointestinal tract, encompassing the small and/or large intestine, as well as the mouth, oesophagus, stomach, and anus (transmural). On the other hand, Ulcerative Colitis is characterized by inflammation limited to the mucosa of the colon, without transmural involvement. Individuals with IBD go through periods of relapse, during which the disease is active, as well as periods of clinical remission. Clinical manifestations of IBD consist of the symptoms such as diarrhoea and/or constipation, the presence of blood or mucus in the stool, and abdominal cramping. Additionally, patients diagnosed with CD may also encounter complications such as bowel obstruction, strictures, and abscess formation.

1.1. Protective mechanisms of the gut

The gastrointestinal tract serves as the principal immune organ within the human body, hosting an impressive 70% of the body's immune cells. Ordinarily, the gastrointestinal tract possesses various protective barriers that effectively hinder the invasion of microbes and other pathogens. These barriers include the mucous lining of the GIT, which possesses the ability to ensure microbes, as well as the epithelial cells that form the external lining of the gastrointestinal tract. These epithelial cells are connected through tight junctions, thereby enhancing their protective capabilities.

Furthermore, the gastrointestinal tract boasts an innate immune system that serves to safeguard its integrity. Remarkably, dendritic cells, akin to colossal kraken, extend tentacle-like protrusions into the mucous layer, enabling them to sample pathogens. These dendritic cells, combined with other innate defenders of the GIT such as macrophages, defences innate lymphoid cells, and IgA antibodies, actively work together to impede the breakthrough of pathogens across the epithelial layer. However, on occasion, those pathogens have the potential to breach the tight junctions and infiltrate the region beneath the epithelium, where they may potentially disseminate throughout the body. In response to this circumstance, the gut adapts by instigating a series of immune responses that encompass B-cells and T-cells. The B-cells possess the ability to transform into active plasma cells, which in turn generate antibodies. These antibodies are capable of attaching themselves to the pathogens and activating T-cells, thereby eliminating these microorganisms.

Consequently, the immune defences of the gut effectively restrain these pathogens, preventing their entry into the body and averting systemic harm. It is of utmost significance to comprehend that the gut must exhibit tolerance towards its own commensal or indigenous microorganisms, which can be facilitated through mechanisms such as the activation of regulatory T-cells. Failure to do so would result in the eradication of the commensal microorganisms by the immune system of the gastrointestinal tract.

2. The role of diet and nutrition in IBD

Diet and nutrition play a pivotal role in managing Inflammatory Bowel Disease (IBD) such as Crohn's disease and ulcerative colitis. Individuals with IBD often face challenges related to nutrient absorption and inflammation, making a carefully tailored diet crucial for symptom alleviation and overall well-being. Identifying trigger foods through a personalized approach and maintaining a well-balanced diet, rich in antioxidants and essential nutrients, can mitigate inflammation and support healing. Collaboration with healthcare professionals, including dietitians, is essential to create an individualized nutrition plan that addresses specific needs and ensures optimal management of IBD symptoms. Regular monitoring and adjustments to the dietary strategy are integral for adapting to the dynamic nature of IBD and optimizing long-term health outcomes.

2.1. Macronutrients and fibre

While there is no clear link between macronutrients and the risk of Inflammatory Bowel Disease (IBD), dietary fiber appears to have a protective effect against Crohn's disease (CD). Increased intake of certain sugars, like sucrose, is associated with a higher risk of ulcerative colitis (UC) and CD. Diets high in saturated fats and monosaccharides, coupled with low fiber, are linked to an elevated risk of CD. The EpiCom cohort study indicates that regular fast-food consumption and high sugar intake are linked to earlier onset, increased disease severity, and a higher likelihood of surgery in UC cases. Although diets high in fructose are associated with metabolic diseases, there is a negative association between fructose intake and IBD risk. Linoleic acid, a dietary n-6 polyunsaturated fatty acid, is linked to increased susceptibility to UC, while substantial consumption of n-3 PUFAs is correlated with a decreased likelihood of developing UC.

Additionally, fermentable carbohydrates, including fermentable oligosaccharides, disaccharides, monosaccharides, and polyols (FODMAPs), represent a category of short-chain carbohydrates poorly absorbed and capable of triggering gastrointestinal symptoms in individuals with quiescent Inflammatory Bowel Disease (IBD). The impact of a low FODMAP diet on IBD patients has been examined and will be explored further. Although there are proven benefits of dietary fiber in maintaining remission, individuals with IBD often express concerns that high-fiber foods can worsen symptoms and believe that their diet may influence the course of their disease. Despite the demonstrated advantages of dietary fiber intake, IBD patients may avoid fiber-rich foods, particularly during active inflammation, citing challenges in digestion.

2.2. Specific carbohydrate diet (SCD)

The Specific Carbohydrate Diet (SCD) is a well-recognized dietary strategy for managing Inflammatory Bowel Disease (IBD). Distinguished by its distinctive composition, the SCD permits the consumption of monosaccharides while excluding disaccharides and most polysaccharides. This highly restrictive diet allows for the intake of fruits and vegetables with higher amylose content, nuts, nut-derived flours, dry-curd cottage cheese, meats, eggs, butter, and various oils. Conversely, it prohibits the consumption of sucrose, maltose, isomaltose, lactose, true and pseudo-grains, grain-derived flours, potatoes, okra, corn, fluid milk, soy, lactose-rich cheeses, and many food additives. Lactose concerns are addressed by incorporating fully fermented yogurt into the diet, ensuring lactose-free status. Grounded in the assimilation of specific carbohydrates requiring minimal digestive processes, the SCD has shown promise in various studies, indicating positive effects on parameters such as anaemia, albumin levels, inflammatory markers, clinical and biochemical aspects, dysbiosis, and the attainment of clinical remission and mucosal healing. However, a thorough scientific evaluation is crucial, given the associated limitations of this dietary approach.

2.3. Anti-inflammatory diet

Derived from the Specific Carbohydrate Diet (SCD), the Inflammatory Bowel Disease Anti-Inflammatory Diet (IBD-AID) was developed by a group associated with the University of Massachusetts Medical School. Originally designed for patients resistant to pharmacological treatments, the IBD-AID aimed to achieve and sustain remission while reducing the frequency and severity of disease exacerbations. However, the effectiveness of this approach fell short of expectations. The IBD-AID comprises five key elements, beginning with the conversion of carbohydrates, including lactose and refined or processed ones, into complex carbohydrates. The second element incorporates the consumption of prebiotics and probiotics, while the third element modifies the intake of dietary fatty acids. The fourth element evaluates the overall dietary pattern, identifying nutrient deficiencies and intolerances. Lastly, the fifth element adjusts food texture through four distinct phases, starting with soft or pureed foods during active flare-ups or as dictated by reported symptoms, with patients progressing to a more comprehensive diet as their symptoms improve.

3. Role of residue in IBD

IBD is a formidable and multifaceted challenge in the realm of gastroenterology and immunology. This group of chronic inflammatory conditions wreaks havoc within the gastrointestinal tract, causing persistent and often debilitating inflammation. Managing IBD involves a multidimensional approach, one facet of which is understanding the influence of dietary residues. These residues encompass a range of undigested food particles and various dietary components of the diet that are not fully broken down or absorbed during the digestive process. They include dietary fibres, complex carbohydrates, and other substances that remain within the digestive system. These dietary residues play a pivotal role in the development and exacerbation of IBD symptoms. The intricate interplay between dietary residues and the gut's immune system can lead to aberrant immune responses and heightened inflammation within the digestive tract. Significantly, the relationship between dietary residues and IBD is not uniform, it is highly individualized, with specific triggers varying from one person to another. The identification and management of specific dietary residues are essential in personalized IBD care, as they can vary widely among individuals and contribute to symptom severity.

3.1. Formation of dietary residues

The journey commencing with the consumption of food involves the initiation of the digestive process. The process commences within the oral cavity where food is subjected to mastication and the actions of enzymes such as amylase, which result in the breakdown of the food into smaller, more manageable fragments. Subsequently, once the ingestion of the food has occurred, it traverses the oesophagus and enters the stomach, an organ where it is met with the presence of stomach acid and additional enzymes that continue the process of breaking down the food.

Nevertheless, it is important to acknowledge that the digestive process is not always concluded in its entirety, and as a result, certain constituents within the diet may remain undigested or unabsorbed within the confines of the stomach and the upper section of the small intestine. These constituents encompass intricate carbohydrates, proteins, fats as well as specific vitamins and minerals. These undigested constituents progress through the intricate network of the digestive system, ultimately arriving at the colon, where they are officially denoted as **dietary residues**.

3.2. Digestion and absorption

In the course of dietary breakdown, the small intestine assumes a vital role in nutrient digestion and absorption. Its remarkable structural design features finger-like projections called villi and even smaller microvilli, significantly amplifying the available surface area for nutrient absorption. During this phase of the digestive process, carbohydrates, proteins, and fats undergo additional transformations.

Carbohydrates, whether derived from grains, fruits, or vegetables, are enzymatically converted into simpler sugars, primarily glucose. Proteins are broken down into their constituent amino acids, while fats are emulsified into fatty acids. Subsequently, these nutrients effortlessly pass through the intestinal lining and reach the circulation. This complex process ensures a consistent supply of energy, essential building blocks for growth and tissue repair, crucial vitamins, minerals, and other necessary components for overall well-being.

Nutrients that evade absorption in the small intestine proceed through the digestive system, advancing to the colon, where they take on the designation of dietary remains. Comprising various undigested elements, these remains engage with the gut microbiota and undergo fermentation in the colon. This interplay between dietary remains and the gut environment holds significance in the context of inflammatory bowel disease (IBD), as it can either contribute to gut health or exacerbate inflammation and related symptoms of IBD. A nuanced understanding of the intricacies of digestion and absorption in the small intestine is crucial for comprehending the impact of dietary remains on the gut environment and the potential development of IBD.

3.3. Types of dietary residues

Dietary Residues encompass a heterogeneous array of dietary constituents that remain undigested and unabsorbed within the body. These remnants manifest in diverse manifestations, reflecting the wide-ranging assortment of dietary components that evade complete digestion and absorption.

Several common manifestations of dietary remnants encompass:

- **Undigested carbohydrates:** Complex carbohydrates, particularly dietary fibre, which can be found in whole grains, fruits, and vegetables, often present challenges in terms of complete digestion.
- **Undigested proteins:** Occasionally, proteins may not be entirely broken down during digestion, leading to the presence of undigested protein fragments.
- **Fats and lipids:** Certain fats, especially long-chain triglycerides, necessitate digestion and emulsification in the small intestine to facilitate absorption. Residues of fats can emerge as a result of malabsorption.

- **Unabsorbed nutrients:** Some vitamins, minerals, and other micronutrients may not undergo full absorption in the small intestine and can consequently contribute to the composition of dietary residues.

The presence of these distinct manifestations of dietary residues underscores the intricate nature of the substances that traverse the digestive system, and eventually play a crucial role in gut health.

3.4. Residues and the gut

Upon reaching the colon, the undigested or unabsorbed components of the diet transform into dietary residues. The colon, a crucial part of the large intestine, assumes responsibility for further processing these residues. It regulates the absorption of water, prepares the material for elimination from the body, and plays a significant role in maintaining the balance of water. In this final stage of the digestive journey, dietary residues can encompass components that are particularly relevant in the context of gastrointestinal health, especially in conditions such as IBD.

Comprehending the formation and composition of dietary residues is of utmost importance, as these residues can interact with the gut microbiota in the colon. The gut microbiota, a complex community of microorganisms residing in the colon, includes bacteria, yeasts, and other microorganisms that are essential for maintaining gut health. Within this environment, certain dietary components, particularly complex carbohydrates like dietary fibre, serve as substrates for fermentation by gut microbiota.

Crucial to processes like fermentation, the interactions between gut microbiota and dietary residues play a central role in breaking down these residues into smaller molecules, resulting in various byproducts, including gases like hydrogen and methane. Among the most significant byproducts of fermentation are short-chain fatty acids (SCFAs), encompassing acetic acid, propionic acid, and butyric acid. Particularly in individuals with Inflammatory Bowel Disease (IBD), these interactions can either contribute to gastrointestinal health or escalate inflammation and worsen symptoms associated with the condition.

3.5. Gut permeability and immune system activation

Gut Permeability, often denoted as “intestinal barrier function” or simply “the gut barrier”, assumes a pivotal role in the maintenance of gut health. This barrier essentially functions as a safeguarding wall encasing our gastrointestinal tract, acting as a discerning gatekeeper that meticulously regulates the transit of substances from our digestive system into the bloodstream, thereby maintaining a delicate equilibrium between the assimilation of vital nutrients and the prevention of harmful substances infiltrating our bodily systems.

The gut barrier predominantly comprises a solitary layer of specialized cells, known as enterocytes, which are intricately interconnected. These enterocytes are held together by intercellular structures referred to as tight junctions, which function akin to impenetrable seals, effectively obstructing the passage of undigested food particles, bacteria, toxins, and other potentially deleterious substances into the bloodstream. Instead, the enterocytes facilitate the passage of absorbed nutrients into the bloodstream, thereby nourishing the body.

Within the context of the gut barrier and its significance in inflammatory bowel disease (IBD), a critical concept surfaces, namely "intestinal permeability". In ordinary circumstances, the gut barrier possesses a degree of permeability, enabling the controlled passage of nutrients while simultaneously excluding unwanted substances. However, in individuals afflicted with IBD and certain other gastrointestinal disorders, this permeability can be compromised.

When the gut barrier becomes "leaky", this signifies a disruption or weakening of the tight junctions connecting the enterocytes. Consequently, the intestinal lining becomes more permeable, allowing indigested residues of dietary intake, harmful bacteria, and their byproducts to traverse the intestinal lining and penetrate the deeper strata of the gut wall.

The phenomenon of "leaky gut" can yield various ramifications:

- **Escalated inflammation:** The presence of dietary residues and bacteria within the deeper layers of the gut wall can incite an immune response, thereby precipitating localized inflammation.
- **Activation of the immune system:** The immune system perceives the foreign substances that have breached the gut barrier as threats, triggering the activation of immune cells and the subsequent release of inflammatory molecules.

- **Chronic inflammation:** In individuals grappling with IBD, this immune response can become chronic, thereby fostering persistent inflammation within the gut.
- **Tissue damage:** Prolonged inflammation can inflict damage upon the gut lining and the adjacent tissues, which serves as a hallmark of IBD.
- **Manifestation of symptoms:** The inflammation and tissue damage within the gut can manifest as the characteristic symptoms associated with IBD, including abdominal pain, diarrhoea, and even more severe complications.

Numerous factors such as genetics, diet, the composition of the gut microbiome, and environmental triggers, all exert their influence on gut permeability.

The interplay between the residual components derived from one's diet and the immune system housed within the gastrointestinal tract, specifically in the milieu of prolonged inflammation, represents a pivotal characteristic in the genesis and intensification of inflammatory responses, immune system mobilization, and structural impairment within the gastrointestinal tract may ultimately culminate in the emergence and advancement of inflammatory bowel disease.

4. The use of biomarkers in the diagnosis of IBD

Researchers have uncovered compelling insights into the pathophysiology of IBD, revealing a pronounced mucosal infiltration of T-cells and plasma cells within the gastrointestinal tract's mucosa. The inflamed gut mucosa's T-cells are responsible for the secretion of inflammatory signalling molecules, known as cytokines, while plasma cells contribute to the production of immunoglobulins, particularly, IgG. This intricate immune response lies at the crux of IBD's complexity.

The gut microenvironment in IBD was found to exhibit a notable departure from the typical balance between pro- and anti-inflammatory cytokines in terms of cytokine profiles. One characteristic that sets this condition apart is the massive abundance of pro-inflammatory cytokines, including interleukin-17, interleukin-23, and tumour necrosis factor-alpha (TNF-alpha). In contrast, there is a noticeable decrease in the amount of anti-inflammatory cytokines like interleukin-10. The protracted inflammatory state that is seen in IBD patients is greatly influenced by this imbalance.

Furthermore, the innate immune defences, inherent to the gastrointestinal tract, also play a crucial role in the pathogenesis of IBD. Innate lymphoid cells, for instance, are acknowledged as active contributors to the inflammatory damage inflicted upon the gut lining, thereby further exacerbating the complexity of the disease.

4.1. Serological antibodies

4.1.1. Perinuclear anti-neutrophil cytoplasmic antibodies (pANCA)

Perinuclear anti-neutrophil cytoplasmic antibodies, demonstrate reactivity towards lysosomal enzymes located within the cytoplasm of neutrophils and monocytes. A specific subset of ANCA targets autoantibodies against neutrophil proteinase 3 (PR3). These PR3-related ANCA have proven valuable as a serological indicator for distinguishing a subset of Inflammatory Bowel Disease (IBD). Serum pANCA has been extensively studied and is recognized for its specificity to Ulcerative Colitis (UC), making it a useful tool for differentiating between UC and Crohn's Disease (CD). It's important to note, however, that while pANCA is specific, its diagnostic utility in accurately identifying patients with suspected UC is somewhat limited by its relatively low sensitivity.

4.1.2. Anti-saccharomyces cerevisiae antibodies (ASCA)

ASCA specifically target the mannan protein in S. cerevisiae. While these antibodies demonstrate notable specificity, they exhibit limited sensitivity in identifying Crohn's Disease (CD) owing to the genetic susceptibility observed in CD patients. ASCA functions as a risk marker for early disease onset and is associated with fibro stenosing and internal-penetrating disease behaviour. However, it is worth noting that the expression of ASCA tends to be relatively diminished among patients with isolated colonic CD.

4.2. C-reactive protein (CRP)

A protein called CRP is produced during the acute phase reaction. It is made up of five identical monomers that are not covalently bound. Its production is carried out by hepatocytes and is initiated by inflammatory cytokines such as TNF-α, IL-1, and IL-1β. Since it has a short half-life, CRP is the most commonly used serum marker to measure inflammation. CRP elevation helps differentiate between mucosal disease that is actively active and IBD that is dormant. A higher CRP concentration and clinical signs of CD correspond to a relapse in the illness. However, CRP is not unique to the illness; higher levels have been seen in conditions such as non-IBD enteritis, inflammatory diseases unrelated to the gastrointestinal system, tissue damage, diabetes, cancer, and cardiovascular disease.

4.3. Biomarkers predicting clinical response

4.3.1. Pro-inflammatory cytokines

Pro-inflammatory cytokines are essential for regulating the inflammatory state of the intestinal microenvironment because they act as signaling molecules that help different immune cells and non-immune cells communicate and coordinate. The idea that these bioactive compounds have significant potential for prognostic value in predicting the therapeutic response to anti-TNF therapy has been supported by multiple lines of empirical investigation.

4.3.2. Vitamin D

Vitamin D, also referred to as 25(OH)D or 25-hydroxyvitamin D, is a modulator of the innate and adaptive immune systems. A lack of this vitamin has been associated with a higher risk of hospitalizations, surgeries, and disease recurrence in patients with inflammatory bowel disease (IBD). In contrast to patients diagnosed with irritable bowel syndrome, individuals with Crohn's disease (CD) demonstrate a greater frequency of vitamin D deficiency and noticeably lower levels of this vitamin.

Moreover, there is a negative correlation between the disease activity in patients with CD and the serum concentration of vitamin D. According to observations, patients who have a vitamin D level below 30 ng/ml are more likely to stop anti-TNF therapy earlier because they do not feel the full therapeutic effect.

References

1. Haskey N, Gibson D. An Examination of Diet for the Maintenance of Remission in Inflammatory Bowel Disease. Nutrients. 2017;9(3):259. doi:10.3390/nu9030259
2. Chiba M, Yoshida T, Komatsu M. From Low-Residue Diets to Plant-Based Diets in Inflammatory Bowel Disease. Dig Dis Sci. 2014;59(12):3129-3130. doi:10.1007/s10620-014-3399-5
3. Loddo I, Romano C. Inflammatory Bowel Disease: Genetics, Epigenetics, and Pathogenesis. Front Immunol. 2015;6. doi:10.3389/fimmu.2015.00551
4. De Castro MM, Pascoal LB, Steigleder KM, et al. Role of diet and nutrition in inflammatory bowel disease. WJEM. 2021;11(1):1-16. doi:10.5493/wjem.v11.i1.1
5. Ahuja A, Pelton M, Raval S, Kesavarapu K. Role of Nutrition in Gastroesophageal Reflux, Irritable Bowel Syndrome, Celiac Disease, and Inflammatory Bowel Disease. Gastro Hep Advances. 2023;2(6):860-872. doi:10.1016/j.gastha.2023.06.010
6. Chen P, Zhou G, Lin J, et al. Serum Biomarkers for Inflammatory Bowel Disease. Front Med. 2020;7:123. doi:10.3389/fmed.2020.00123
7. Kang Y, Park H, Choe BH, Kang B. The Role and Function of Mucins and Its Relationship to Inflammatory Bowel Disease. Front Med. 2022;9:848344. doi:10.3389/fmed.2022.848344

8. Shivashankar R, Lewis JD. The Role of Diet in Inflammatory Bowel Disease. Curr Gastroenterol Rep. 2017;19(5):22. doi:10.1007/s11894-017-0563-z
9. Jones JL, Foxx-Orenstein AE. The Role of Probiotics in Inflammatory Bowel Disease. Dig Dis Sci. 2007;52(3):607-611. doi:10.1007/s10620-006-9225-y

8.

Lactose Intolerance and Inflammatory Bowel Disease: A Comprehensive Overview

S. Shobana[1]*, M. Narmadha[2], S.G. Nandhika Jothi[2]

[1]Department of Biotechnology, Vel Tech Rangarajan Dr. Sagunthala R&D Institute of Science and Technology, Avadi-600062, Tamil Nadu.

[2] Department of Biotechnology, Prathyusha Engineering College, Tiruvallur 602025, Tamil Nadu

Email: shobidhilip89@gmail.com

Abstract

Lactose intolerance and inflammatory bowel disease (IBD), specifically Crohn's disease, are substantial gastrointestinal disorders with a notable global health impact. Lactose intolerance stems from insufficient lactase enzyme activity, resulting in ineffective digestion of lactose, a prevalent sugar found in dairy products. Its prevalence is widespread, affecting a noteworthy portion of the world population. Crohn's disease and other forms of inflammatory bowel disease are chronic inflammatory illnesses that primarily affect the digestive tract and are characterized by periods of remission interspersed with flare-ups. These gastrointestinal ailments profoundly influence an individual's well-being and necessitate effective management strategies. This thorough chapter aims to explore the intricate correlation between lactose intolerance and inflammatory bowel disease. It delves into their epidemiology, root etiological factors, clinical presentations, and the latest advancements in diagnostic methods. Additionally, it looks into possible connections between lactose intolerance and inflammatory bowel disease patients' symptoms getting worse. Grasping this complex interplay is vital for devising customized treatment plans, minimizing discomfort, and enhancing the overall quality of life for affected individuals. The chapter underscores the importance of dietary alterations, especially lactose reduction, in alleviating symptoms for individuals dealing with both lactose intolerance and inflammatory bowel disease. Tailored dietary interventions and the integration of innovative therapeutic approaches are essential to achieve optimal outcomes for individuals navigating the intricate relationship between lactose intolerance and inflammatory bowel disease. A profound comprehension of these disorders is crucial for clinicians, researchers, and affected individuals, offering the potential for more effective management and an improved quality of life within this challenging health landscape.

1. Introduction

Today, digestive issues are widespread and frequent. Lactase deficiency varies among different ethnic groups, affecting around 15% of people with northern European ancestry, up to 80% of Latinos and Black people, and nearly 100% of American Indians and Asians. Those with lactose intolerance exhibit a diverse spectrum of lactose malabsorption levels, with most of them being able to drink up to 12 ounces of milk every day without encountering any symptoms(*Swagerty Jr et.al,2002)(Lomer et.al,2008,).*Since their first contemporary descriptions are some 75–100 years ago, the inflammatory bowel disorders (IBDs), which are mostly represented by ulcerative colitis and Crohn's disease also include noninfectious inflammations of the colon, which have both baffled gastroenterologists and immunologists *(Strober et.al,2007)*lactose intolerance and inflammatory bowel disease are briefly described in this chapter. Both have major issues, and the majority of people are affected by them. Clinical research's major goal is to treat various digestive illnesses and find a treatment for all of them. Most digestive illnesses lack a proper cause or justification for occurrence. It lacks an accurate diagnosis. Here are two illnesses: inflammatory bowel disease and lactose intolerance. Let's examine its consequences, symptoms, diagnosis and treatment.

2. Lactose intolerance

The enzyme lactase gets converted into lactose into glucose and galactose*(Büller et.al,1990),* they are then digested in the small intestine. Lactose intolerance develops when this procedure is unproductive in breaking down lactose. Over 30 million Americans suffer from lactose intolerance*(Johnsonet.al,1993)* which is more common among Asian, American, and African populations. There are four types of lactose intolerance: primary, secondary, congenital, and developmental. Primary lactose intolerance, also referred to as adult hypolactasia, afflicts approximately 70% of the global population, with the majority hailing from Asian, African, and Hispanic ethnic backgrounds. It begins between the ages of 5-7 and becomes most apparent between the ages of 30 and 40. In Europe, the incidence drops significantly and reaches only 5% in places like Switzerland and Denmark*(Campbell et.al,2005)*.In Europe, the prevalence varies, roughly with 50% of responders being above the age of 60. The combination of Crohn's disease and celiac disease, as well as other illnesses, injuries, microbial infections and surgeries, might result in secondary lactose intolerance*(Bhatnagar et.al,2007)*.One major aspect that might influence how the at-risk infant's illness progresses (e.g., less than 3 months or malnourished) is lactose intolerance*(Heyman et.al,2006)*. Congenital lactose intolerance is an inherited condition that results in severe digestive problems and diarrhea. It is widespread among communities in Northern Europe, Scandinavia, Holland, Spain, Italy and Arab nations who practice pastoralism. It is about 1% in Asia and Africa. Proteins are shortened by frame shifts or mutations that missense in the LPH coding region*(Amiri et.al,2015)* which is the underlying cause of this condition. In a study encompassing 32 individuals, researchers identified five different mutations within the LCT coding region. Remarkably, one of these mutations appeared in a homozygous state in 84% of the instances. Developmental lactose intolerance is marked by reduced lactase levels, a condition stemming from preterm birth typically occurring between weeks 28 to 32 of gestation. Interestingly, fetal lactase enzyme activity rises after week 34 and ranges its zenith at the time of birth*(Arora&singhala,2011)*.Following weaning, approximately two-thirds of the global population experience a genetically predetermined reduction in lactase production, which is referred to as primary lactase insufficiency. Furthermore, secondary lactase deficiency can manifest in individuals with lactase persistence due to factors such as gastrointestinal infections, abdominal surgery, inflammatory bowel disease, and various other medical conditions. Both diseases must be separated from deficiency in congenital lactase, a very rare infantile illness that is described in around 40 cases, mostly in Finland.

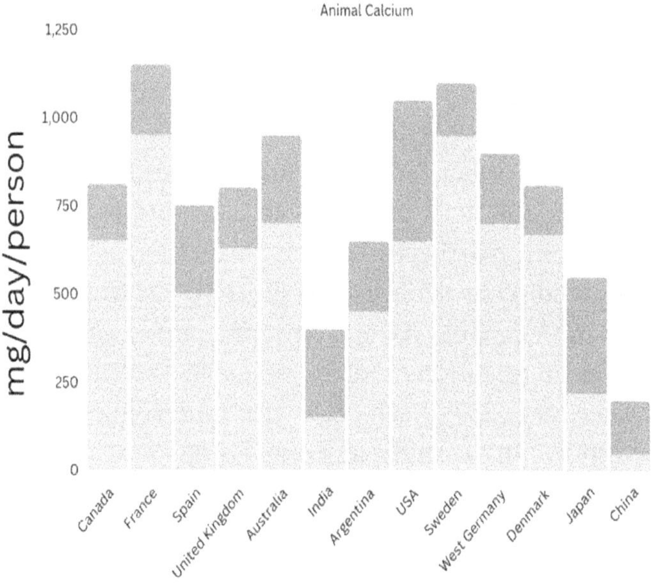

Diagram (1): Survey of Lactose intolerance

3. Mechanism

Lactase-phlorizin hydrolase, is a protein that is found on the brush boundary of intestinal villi, particularly abundant in the mid-jejunum, extends as finger-like protrusions. These structures serve to amplify the overall surface area of the small intestine, enhancing its capacity to absorb various substrates. This protein acts a vital role in the digestion of lactose within the small intestine. Lactose is hydrolyzed and broken down into simpler sugars like glucose and galactose by this enzyme. The right absorption depends on the jejunum mucosa's enzyme activity and transit time. Absence of the lactase enzyme prevents absorption from happening. This process leads to the influx of fluid into the gut lumen, which has an osmolality three times higher than that of sugar and disrupts the electrochemical balance between the blood and the gut contents. Lactose that remains unabsorbed proceeds into the colon, where it undertakes digestion by bacteria, that results in the formation of short-chain fatty acids and gases (CO_2, CH_4, H_2)(*Vandenplas, Y. 2015)(Campbell et.al,2010)*. These byproducts may result in various gastrointestinal symptoms. Furthermore, alike biological processes affect other fermentable oligosaccharides, polyols (FODMAPs) monosaccharides and disaccharides that are poorly absorbed. It also results in cleavage of monosaccharides. Colonic mucosa cannot absorb this monosaccharide. This raises the osmotic and fluid pressure in the bowel *(Swagerty Jr et.al, 2002)*.

4. Symptoms

In general, symptoms of lactose intolerance tend to manifest only when lactase activity drops below the 50% threshold. Regular consumption of lactose could also have an impact. Although consuming lactose does not increase lactase expression, gut flora adaptation may be able to promote tolerance. In a randomized crossover study, scientists investigated the gastrointestinal symptoms in 30 individuals with severe lactose intolerance. These participants reported experiencing symptoms after consuming less than 240 ml of milk. The group had an average oldness of 29.4 years, with ages that range from 18 to 50.

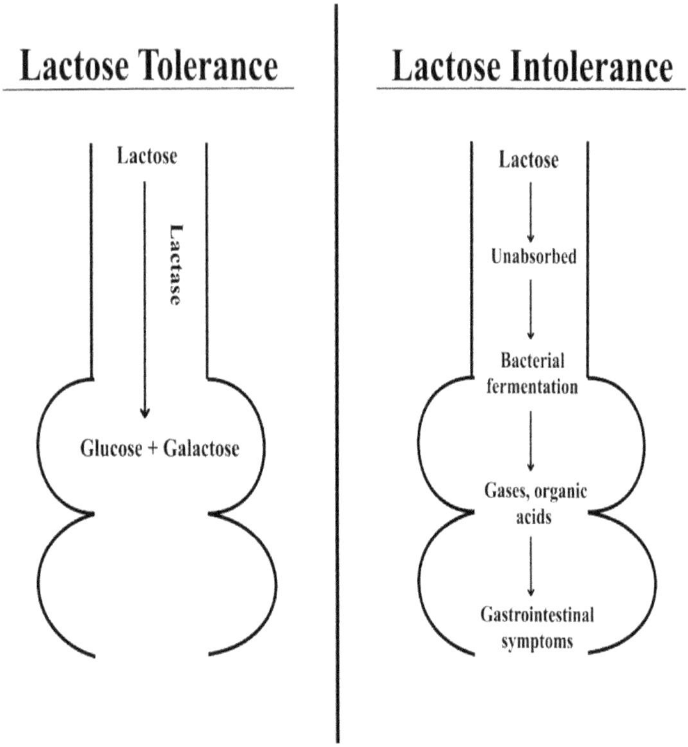

Diagram (2): Mechanism of Lactose intolerance

Among them, nine individuals reserved the ability to digest lactose, while the 21 had lactose malabsorption. Among the group of 21 participants with lactose malabsorption, there were eight men and thirteen women, with an average age of 29.4 years. The racial composition was as follows: eight were of white ethnicity, five were Hispanic, seven were Asian, and one was of black ethnicity. Notably, the majority of these individuals experienced minimal digestive symptoms, with average symptom-severity ratings for symptoms like bloating, diarrhea, stomach pain, and flatus ranging from 0.1 to 1.2. Furthermore, there were no reports of vomiting or diarrhea among the participants*(Suarez, F. L et.al,1995)*.Due to an inability to digest and absorb milk sugars, people with lactose intolerance have symptoms including bloating, cramps, diarrhea, gas, and borborygmi*(He et.al,2008)*.Based on the degree of lactose intolerance and the quantity of lactose taken, the symptoms might change.

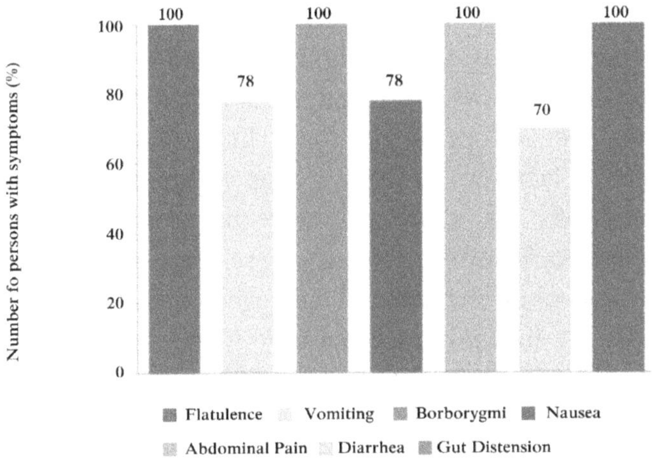

Diagram (3): Symptoms of lactose intolerance

The signs and symptoms include anorexia, diarrhea, vomiting, stomach noises, pain, swelling, flatulence, and constipation. Headache, memory loss, musculoskeletal pain, irregular heartbeat, dry mouth, depression, oral mucosal ulcers, and other allergic reactions are examples of non-intestinal symptoms *(Silberman et.al,2019)*.Lactose intolerance affects about 20% of the people. Due to environmental factors or the co-occurrence of other digestive issues, people who assert that they are lactose intolerant frequently suffer from a condition known as the "nocebo effect".

5. Diagnosis

The milk test for suppression and provocation is a diagnostic test involving the elimination of lactose from the diet for about two weeks, followed by the reintroduction of lactose. If symptoms manifest upon reintroduction, it is indicative of lactose intolerance in the individual *(Vesa et.al, 2008)*.If the symptoms go away, the person is not lactose intolerant. The biggest drawback of this diagnosis is that it is impossible to identify asymptomatic lactose intolerance. A jejunal sample's lactase activity was directly measured biochemically as the first step in identifying lactose maldigestion. Due to its invasiveness, endoscopic duodenal biopsy has taken the place of this procedure. Despite a 40% decrease in mean lactase activity in the duodenum, the Quick lactase test which is used to diagnose severe duodenal hypolactasia on postbulbar duodenum samples was effective with 95% sensitivity and 100% specificity, respectively *(Mattar, R et.al, 2012)*blood Glucose levels was measured before and after the consumption of an oral dose of lactose at specified time breaks is another method for evaluating lactose tolerance. An increase in blood glucose levels of no more than 20 mg/dL is regarded as a sign of lactose tolerance (*INTOLERANCE, P. L. 1978)*.Nevertheless, of all the indirect lactose tolerance trials that are now on the market, taking a breath hydrogen test after consuming 50 g of lactose was deemed to be the best useful test for lactase deficiency screening in the general population. The utility of this technique in therapeutic settings is still under study*(Di Rienzo et.al, 2013)*.The identification of lactase-persistence alleles has enabled genetic testing for lactase non-persistence using a range of techniques, restriction fragment length polymorphism that includes real-time polymerase chain reaction and Pyrosequencing technology*(Shaw et.al,1999)*.The genetic test is a straightforward, non-invasive, and simpler investigation than the lactose hydrogen breath test. Stool acidity test is when unabsorbed carbohydrates are broken down by bacteria and volatile fatty acids are produced. This lowers pH by 5.5, and persons who are lactose intolerant generate acidic stools. The pH of an infant's feces is lower in breastfed babies*(Arola et.al, 1994)*.As a result, breastfeeding babies cannot use this method. The lactose hydrogen breath test is regarded as the recognized test for diagnosing lactose malabsorption.

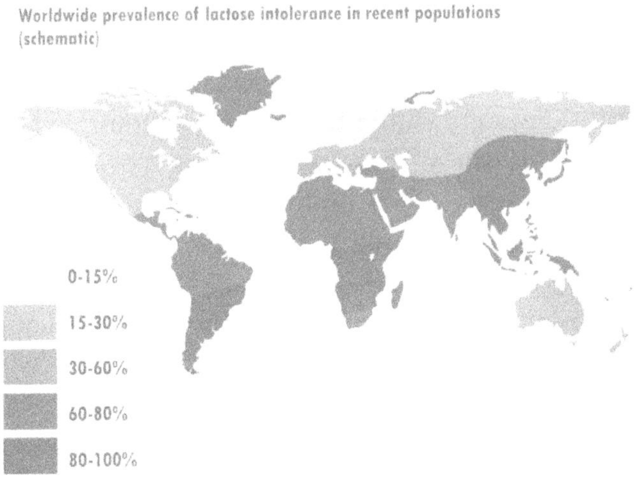

Diagram (4): Prevalence of lactose intolerance

6. Treatment

Treatment for lactose intolerance includes reducing or eliminating lactose intakereplacing it with other foods, using enzyme substitutes or lactase supplements *(Catanzaro et.al,2021).* A further key approach for hydrolyzing lactose is enzyme supplementation treatment using lactase from nonhuman sources *(Roxas,M,2008)*Exogenous lactase has the capability to catalyze the hydrolysis of lactose into glucose and galactose, thereby improving its absorption. It is derived from *Aspergillus oryzae* or *Kluyveromyces lactis.* Using the lactose breath test, 22% of the 96 persons who were given lactase supplements completely normalized, whereas 18% were completely non-responsive. The patient has the option of purchasing or making milk with less lactose by incubating regular milk with a lactase preparation overnight. Although this type of treatment has the benefit of being accessible whenever a food containing lactose is consumed, the cost of lactase tablets drives up the price of milk by between 150% and 300%*(Wilt et.al,2010).*Fermented milk products are proven to help lactose maldigesters with intolerance symptoms and lactose digestion. This study showed that plain yogurt from the store works just as well as prehydrolyzed milk to lower H2 levels and relieve symptoms. The presence of endogenous lactase activity in the bacteria used to ferment yogurt explains its utility in lactose digestion. The production of yogurt typically involves milk being cultured with *L. bulgaricus* and *S. thermophilus*, both of which are lactic acid bacteria. Both during fermentation processes and after lactose consumption, these bacteria take role in lactose breakdown. Fermentation is estimated to reduce the lactose content of food by 25–50% *(Suarez et.al,1995)*.Current recommendations no longer advise entities with lactose intolerance to completely avoid all dairy related products. In fact, the majority of lactose intolerant individuals can safely consume around 12 to 15 grams of lactose daily without experiencing significant symptoms*(Catanzaro et.al,2006)*. In comparison to skimmed milk and aqueous lactose solution, full-fat milk, often referred to as high-energy milk, improves lactose tolerance. This is attributed to the reported effect of fat on enhancing carbohydrate absorption. Fat accomplishes this by slowing down intestinal transit and stomach emptying, which, in turn, extends the duration that enzymes remain in contact with their substrate. Lactose replacement treatment is also utilized to convert lactose into glucose and galactose. After four weeks, probiotics can help to reduce hydrogen production, which can aid with lactose intolerance*(Szilagyi et,al.1994)*.Delactosation is a procedure that either completely eliminates or drastically decreases the lactose content in milk. There are two methods to accomplish this: the first involves the use of the enzyme galactosidase to hydrolyze lactose into glucose and galactose, and the second entails ultrafiltration combined with a reduction in lactase enzyme content*(Szilagyi et.al,2018)*.Temperature control is essential for minimizing bacterial flora during the process, which takes about 15 to 20 hours at a temperature of 6 to 10 ^{0}C. This approach has an 85% success rate depending on the rate of lactose hydrolysis. This process is termed as lacteal products because it also eliminates salts and necessitates additional product modification. Lactose-free milk or dairy products are produced using delactosation.

7. Chron's Disease (Cd)

The name "Chron's" is derived from an American gastroenterologist Burrill Bernard Chron who made a first study and identified about this disease was later named after him. Any area of the digestive system from the mouth to the anus can be impacted by Chron's disease, a chronic inflammatory bowel illness. It is characterized by inflammation that lasts deep into the layers of bowel tissue, which frequently gives symptoms like severe abdominal pain, diarrhoea and fatigue*(Petagna wt.al,2020).*

7.1. Mechanism of Chron's Disease

Pathogenesis and Inflammation:

Chronic inflammation brought on by the immune system's reaction to bacterial antigens is known as Crohn's disease, and it is impacted by natural defensive mechanisms such as the release of intestinal mucus.It is sustained by cell interaction with integrins, adhesion molecules, and chemokines, leading to elevated levels of inflammatory cytokines. Leucocyte MAcCAM-1, CD44, CD26, and MMPs play crucial roles. Interleukins expression, which regulate immune cell maturation and growth, is anomalous in CD patients*(Shanahan et.al,2002).*

7.2. Genetic studies and chron's disease

Studies on twins and families have revealed a strong hereditary impact on the development of chronic kidney disease (CD). CARD15, ATG16L1, IBD5 locus and IRGM.The IL-23 receptor have all been discovered as unique genetic loci. However, because of their limited penetrance, these polymorphisms cannot be considered causal.

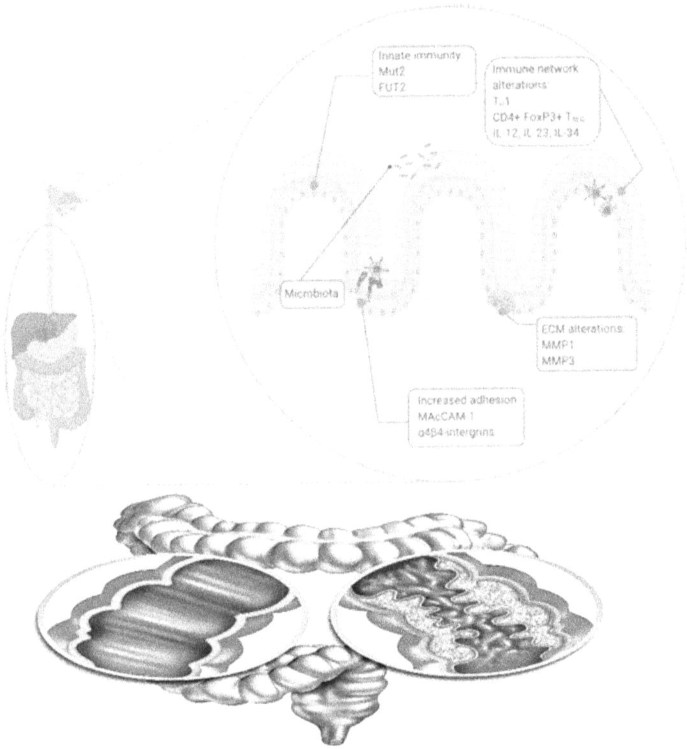

Diagram (5): Immuno-mediated pathogenesis of Chron's disease

For instance, given a chosen group of 100,000 people, approximately fifteen thousand would be classified as heterozygous for one version of CARD15, and about 500 would be homozygous or compound heterozygous. Of those that develop CD, only 28 have CARD15 polymorphisms and 28 of them are simple or compound heterozygous. Genetic risk factors are insufficiently thorough, leading to missing heritability. Phenotypic abnormalities are common in CD patients, potentially leading to mucosal barrier failure or inflammation*(Shanahan, F. 2002).*

7.3. Stages of immunopathogenesis pathway

Stage 1: Penetration of luminal contents into the bowel wall

Remission is induced by redirecting the faecal stream, while recurrence is triggered by returning ileostomy run-off into the excluded ileum. To develop CD lesions, the fecal stream must get past the intestinal barrier. Gut epithelial cells form an impermeable barrier to luminal contents, which is covered with mucus composed of mucin glycoproteins and defensins*(L, Neurath MF.2015)*immunoglobulins, and other substance. Enterocytes, lymphocytes, and other cells emit these chemical compounds. Studies indicate increased intestinal permeability in people with chronic intestinal inflammation (CD), but the underlying mechanism is unknown. This porosity may predict recurrence in macroscopically normal smaller bowels, lending credence to the hypothesis that increased permeability is the major initiating cause. According to studies, typical relatives and spouses of CD patients have higher permeability, suggesting environmental and genetic triggers. This makes the mucosa more vulnerable to harm, with weaker mucosa having lower resistance. Other environmental elements could also have a role. Mucin genes like MUC19 increase the risk of colitis, possibly due to damage to the mucous membrane and mutations in mucin production, PTGE4R, and inflammation.

Stage 2: Impaired excretory excrement removal from the colon wall

A lower concentration of acute inflammatory agents such as IL-8 and IL-1 at cutaneous windows and injured gut mucosa impairs neutrophil accumulation in CD patients. The majority of the body's resident macrophages, which are replenished by monocytes from the peripheral bloodstream in the colon, emit cytokines that cause inflammation *(Sewell, G. W,2009)*.In the aftermath of stimulation with heat-killed, macrophages from CD patients released considerably fewer cytokines that were pro-inflammatory. It is therefore unlikely that the results were caused by persistent inflammation in the bowel, which is supported by the distinct cytokine profiles observed in macrophages grown in individuals with UC. It was predicted that delayed the proliferation of neutrophil would impair the permission of intestinal contents, facilitating bacteria to gain possession of bowel tissues. Chronic granulation disease (CGD), a lack of immunity disorder caused by oxidase gene mutations, frequently causes bowel irritation that can be distinct from CD. These flaws cause these patients to have a significantly decreased ability to remove foreign material, which naturally makes them more prone to CD. In CARD15 wild-type CD patients, exogenous MDP was discovered to repair an anomaly within neutrophil formation, an ability that had been impeded by an abundance of CD-associated polymorphisms. Variants in the CARD15 sequence may also be associated with altered production of anti-inflammatory cytokines by PBMCs and decreased expression of alpha defensin by Paneth cells, suggesting that NOD2 may be involved in several phases of CD pathogenesis. The concept that the clearance of foreign material plays a crucial role in the progression of bowel inflammation is supported by the defective autophagy and pathogen expulsion caused by CD-associated ATG16L1 mutations and functional inhibition of ATG16L1 or IRGM. Patients with CD should be more vulnerable to bacterial infection if the disease is brought on by a systemic deficiency in innate immunity.

Stage 3: Adaptive immune responses that compensate

When there is no recruitment of neutrophils, macrophages ingest uncleared material and produce granulomata. T cells are drawn to pro-inflammatory cytokines and chemokines, which polarize them to the Th1 phenotype—a stage of chronic inflammation that is different from the first acute response. The CD is a long-term intestinal inflammation that is distinguished by a high cell turnover rate and the exposure of antigens to the immune system. It is typified by systemic reactions and local tissue injury, with lymphocyte infiltration and granuloma development serving as compensatory measures. The CD does not fit Witebsky's criteria for what constitutes an autoimmune disease*(Shanahan, F. (2002)(L, Neurath,2015).*

7.4. Diagnosis

Surgical indications for Chron's disease:

The contrast of various anatomical positions is used to analyze information gathered from 500 patients with Chron's disease who went through surgery. (1) ileocolic-225 patients; (2) small intestinal-130 patients; (3) colonic-127 patients; (4) anorectal- 18 patients.

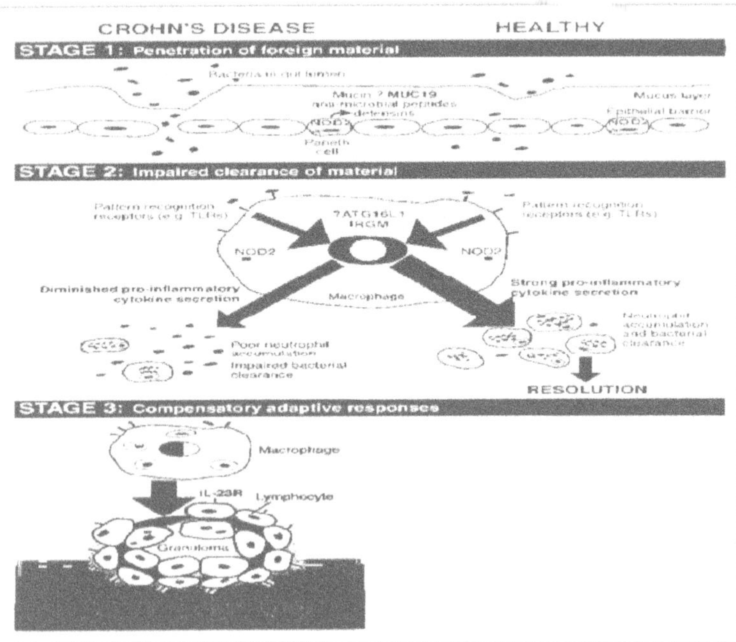

Diagram (6): Immunopathogenesis pathway

TABLE 1. Surgery should be considered in patients who have an ileocolic pattern.

INDICATIONS	No. of patients 1966-1969	No. of patients 1972-1973	Total	%
Perianal disease	22	6	28	12
Internal fistula and abscess	56	42	98	44
Toxicmegalacon	5	0	5	2

Poor response to medical therapy	9	6	15	7
Intestinal obstruction	54	25	79	35
total	146	79	225	

TABLE 2. Indication for surgery amid patients with S1n4l/ intestinal pattern

INDICATIONS	No.of patients 1966-1969	No.of patients 1972-1973	Total	%
Perianal disease	6	0	6	5
Internal fistula and abscess	24	17	41	32
Intestinal obstruction	45	27	72	55
Toxic megalacon	0	3	11	9
Poor response to medical therapy	8	3	11	9
total	87	47	103	

TABLE 3. The surgical indications in patients with a colonic pattern

INDICATIONS	No.of patients 1966-1969	No.of patients 1972-1973	Total	Percentage

Perianal disease	17	6	24	19
Internal fistula and abscess	19	11	30	23
Intestinal obstruction	9	6	15	12
Toxic megalacon	14	11	25	20
Poor response to medical therapy	16	17	33	26
total	75	52	127	

7.5 Complications

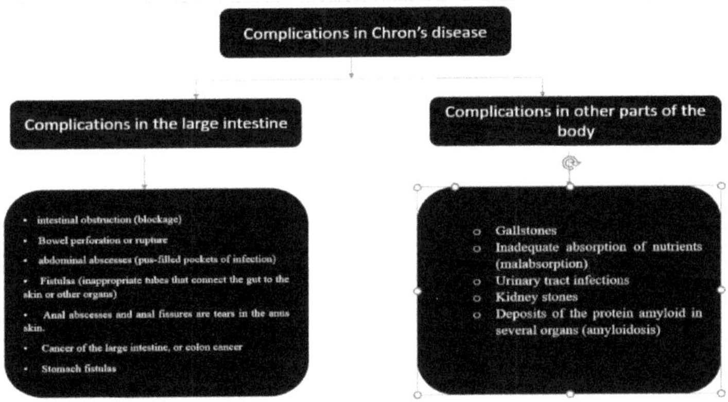

Diagram (6); Complications of Chron's disease

7.6 Treatment

Treatment for Crohn's disease using corticosteroids and corticotrophin

Thirty individuals got anti-tuberculosis therapy in addition to corticotrophin or corticosteroids, seven patients received both forms of treatment concurrently, and one patient received both at different times. A number of the histological similarities between Crohn's illness and tuberculosis lesions, anti-tuberculous medication was given as a pilot trial at a particular time. The two groups were studied separately*(D'Haens et.al,1998).*

TABLE 1: The diagnostic criteria employed in patient selection.

Criteria for diagnosis	**Number of patients**
Histology characteristic of Chron's disease	54
Histology compatible with Chron's disease	18
Typical clinical picture,radiological;non-specific histology	7
Typical clinical picture,radiological;no histology	26

TABLE 2: Distribution of disease

Distribution of disease	**All cases**	**Treat with A.C.T.H orvcorticosteriods**	
		Alone	**With anti-tuberculosis drugs**
Extensive small bowel	12	30	0

Ileo-caecal	56	30	2
Ileo-colic	27	30	5
colon	10	30	10
Total	105	30	7

TABLE 3. Latter course in individuals who, while receiving corticotrophin or corticosteroids without anti-tuberculous therapy, initially showed recovery.

Distribution of disease	Number with initial responses	No further treatment	Continuing treatmnet	resection	Died
Extensive small bowel	4	3	7	0	1
Ileo-caecal	3	3	7	0	0
Ileo-colic	7	3	7	2	1
colon	8	3	7	6	2
Total	22	3	7	8	4

8. Ulcerative Collitis

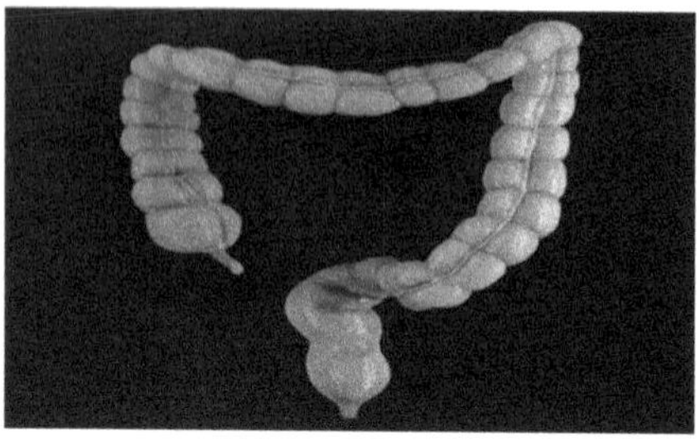

Diagram (7): ulcerative colitis

8.1. Types of ulcerative collitis *(Gajendran,m et.al, 2019)*

- Ulcerative proctitis happens when the inflammation is limited to the region closest to the anus, which is also referred to as the rectum. The only indication of the illness could involve rectal bleeding.
- Proctosigmoiditis: Swelling of the lower end of the colon, the sigmoid colon, and the abdomen. The symptoms include bloody diarrhea, abdominal cramps, and an inability to pass gas despite strong cravings.
- •Left-sided colitis: The sigmoid gland, descending colon, and the rectum are all affected by inflammation. The indications and symptoms include bloody diarrhea, left-sided stomach cramps, and the urge to urinate.
- Pancolitis: This kind usually affects every part of the colon and results in severe cramping and bleeding in the abdomen, exhaustion, and substantial weight loss.

It is unknown what specifically causes ulcerative colitis. Stress and diet have been suspected earlier. Researchers understand that while these factors are not linked to ulcerative colitis, they can exacerbate the condition. One potential reason could be an immune system failure. Your immune system attacks digestive tract cells in an attempt to neutralize an invasive virus or bacteria, but this is offset by an imbalanced defense. It seems that having family members with ulcerative colitis increases the likelihood of developing the illness, which is another indication that heredity may be involved*(Langan, R. C et.al,2007)*.Nonetheless, this family history is uncommon in the majority of ulcerative colitis sufferers.

8.2. Diagnosis

Patients and methods

The data comprises people living in Copenhagen County who had Crohn's disease or ulcerative colitis between 1960 and 1978. Diagnostic criteria were published using endoscopy, X-rays, and histology/cytology findings. 186 patients—783 with ulcerative colitis and 185 with Crohn's disease—were included in the study. Data was collected prospectively from diagnosis in our department (695 patients), and 28% from four other Copenhagen hospitals, preparing a retrospective study. The study searched Copenhagen general practitioners and specialists for inflammatory bowel disease cases, finding only eight patients (~1%). Due to insufficient clinical data, these patients were excluded. Data processing and statistical evaluation involved chi-square tests and multiple Poisson models.

Table I. Age at diagnosis

	MEDIAN YEARS	RANGE YEARS
ULCERATIVE COLITIS, NO=783	33.8 F:34.4;M:33.0	2-87
CHRON'S DISEASE NO=185	33.3 F:33.3;M:33.3	4-76

From 1960 and 1978, 783 patients were diagnosed with ulcerative colitis, with 342 male (44%) and 441 female (56%). Table I shows the material's age distribution. The average age at diagnosis was identical for both sexes.

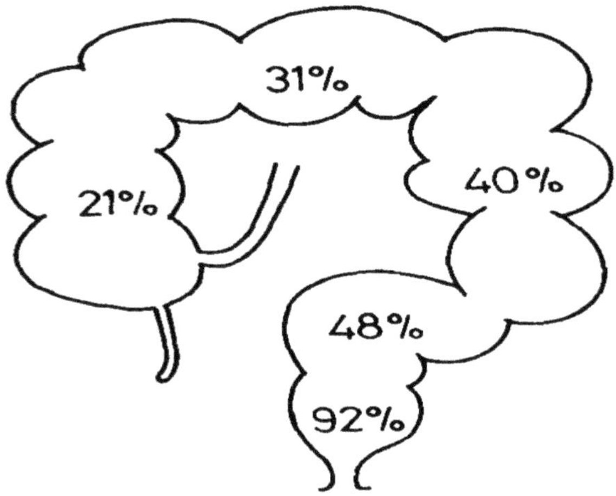

Diagram (8): Localization at diagnosis in 783 patients with ulcerative colitis

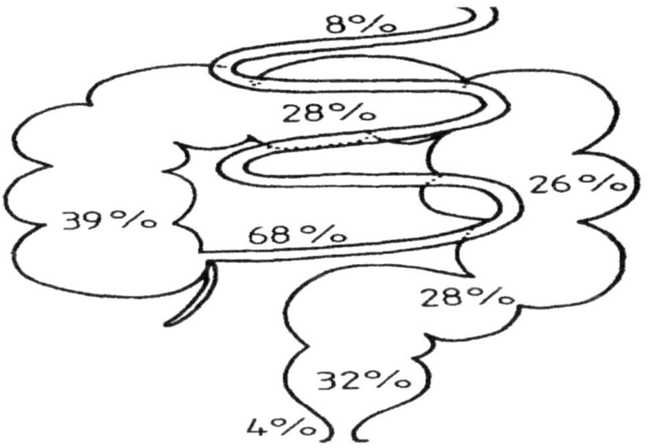

Diagram (9) Localization at diagnosis in 185 patients with Crohn's disease.

8.3. Treatment

Management of active UC

The diagnostic workup for UC includes clinical evaluation, medical history, full blood count, ESR, stool microbiology, CRP, ultrasound, and endoscopy. If doubt arises, endoscopic and histological confirmation should be repeated. Treatment depends on activity, distribution, disease course, relapse frequency, extraintestinal manifestations, previous medications, and patient preferences (*DeRoche et.al,2014)*

Severe UC

Severe UC, *(Farmeret.al,1976)*characterized by more than 6 bloody stools each day and systemic involvement, requires intensive treatment and surveillance. Intravenous steroids are the main therapy, and patient's refractory to oral treatment can give a certain the tumor necrosis factor blocker IFX at 5 mg/kg. Colectomy rates in severe UC patients needing intravenous corticosteroids can be as high as 29%. Patients should be offered to the colorectal surgeon on admission and provided daily care to avoid delays. Colectomy should be discussed if worsening condition or lack of improvement after 3 days of steroid treatment.

9. Future treatment for UC and medications

In patients with severe UC, colectomy rates vary from 15% to 29%, requiring intravenous corticosteroids. For treatment, alternative therapies like ova, nicotine, and omega-3 fatty acids have emerged. Oral ova have been revealed to be effective in remission in 43% of patients, while nicotine has been shown to be considered effective in active UC. However, no direct equivalent trials with omega-3 fatty acids have been conducted *(Janowitz H. D et,al,1975)*. TNF-AB preparations such as certolizumab, etanercept, and adalimumab, which could be approved for UC treatment this year, are among the advances in biological therapy. Other biologicals have been tested for individuals with acute steroid-refractory UC *(Meier, J &Sturum,A.2017)(H., Torp-Pedersen et.al,1983)*.

10. Conclusions

This chapter concludes that there isn't a cure to boost your body's lactase production, but symptom management is possible through dietary adjustments. While individuals with lactose intolerance were traditionally advised to steer clear of dairy products, modern health experts recommend experimenting with various dairy foods to identify those causing fewer symptoms. IBD cannot be cured; however, there are periods of remission when the disease is inactive.

Medications can help decrease inflammation and extend the duration of these remission periods, but a definitive cure does not currently exist. Inflammatory bowel disease and lactose intolerance can only be treated; they cannot be fully healed. Treatments can only slow down the activity; they cannot stop it.

References

1. Swagerty Jr, D. L., Walling, A. D., & Klein, R. M. (2002). Lactose intolerance. American family physician, 65(9), 1845-1851.
2. Lomer, M. C., Parkes, G. C., & Sanderson, J. D. (2008). lactose intolerance in clinical practice–myths and realities. Alimentary pharmacology & therapeutics, 27(2), 93-103.
3. Strober, W., Fuss, I., & Mannon, P. (2007). The fundamental basis of inflammatory bowel disease. The Journal of clinical investigation, 117(3), 514-521.
4. Büller, H. A., & Grand, R. J. (1990). Lactose intolerance. Annual review of Medicine, 41(1), 141-148.
5. Johnson, A. O., Semenya, J. G., Buchowski, M. S., Enwonwu, C. O., & Scrimshaw, N. S. (1993). Correlation of lactose maldigestion, lactose intolerance, and milk intolerance. The American journal of clinical nutrition, 57(3), 399-401.
6. Campbell, A. K., Waud, J. P., & Matthews, S. B. (2005). The molecular basis of lactose intolerance. Science progress, 88(3), 157-202.
7. Bhatnagar, S., & Aggarwal, R. (2007). Lactose intolerance. Bmj, 334(7608), 1331-1332.

8. Heyman, M. B., & Committee on Nutrition. (2006). Lactose intolerance in infants, children, and adolescents. Pediatrics, 118(3), 1279-1286.
9. Amiri, M., Diekmann, L., von Köckritz-Blickwede, M., & Naim, H. Y. (2015). The diverse forms of lactose intolerance and the putative linkage to several cancers. Nutrients, 7(9), 7209-7230.
10. Arora, S., & Singla, N. LACTOSE INTOLERANCE IN INFANTS, CHILDREN, AND ADOLESCENTS. age, 7, 8.
11. Vandenplas, Y. (2015). Lactose intolerance. Asia Pacific journal of clinical nutrition, 24(Supplement).
12. Campbell, A. K., Matthews, S. B., Vassel, N., Cox, C. D., Naseem, R., Chaichi, J., ... & Wann, K. T. (2010). Bacterial metabolic 'toxins': a new mechanism for lactose and food intolerance, and irritable bowel syndrome. Toxicology, 278(3), 268-276.
13. Swagerty Jr, D. L., Walling, A. D., & Klein, R. M. (2002). Lactose intolerance. American family physician, 65(9), 1845-1851.
14. Suarez, F. L., Savaiano, D. A., & Levitt, M. D. (1995). A comparison of symptoms after the consumption of milk or lactose-hydrolyzed milk by people with self-reported severe lactose intolerance. New England Journal of Medicine, 333(1), 1-4.
15. He, T., Venema, K., Priebe, M. G., Welling, G. W., Brummer, R. J., & Vonk, R. J. (2008). The role of colonic metabolism in lactose intolerance. European journal of clinical investigation, 38(8), 541-547.
16. Silberman, E. S., & Jin, J. (2019). Lactose intolerance. JAMA, 322(16), 1620-1620.

17. Vesa, T. H., Marteau, P., & Korpela, R. (2000). Lactose intolerance. Journal of the American College of Nutrition, 19(sup2), 165S-175S
18. Mattar, R., de Campos Mazo, D. F., & Carrilho, F. J. (2012). Lactose intolerance: diagnosis, genetic, and clinical factors. Clinical and experimental gastroenterology, 113-121.
19. INTOLERANCE, P. L. (1978). The practical significance of lactose intolerance in children. Pediatrics, 62(2).
20. Di Rienzo, T., D'angelo, G., D'aversa, F., Campanale, M. C., Cesario, V., Montalto, M., ... & Ojetti, V. (2013). Lactose intolerance: from diagnosis to correct management. European Review for Medical & Pharmacological Sciences, 17.
21. Di Rienzo, T., D'angelo, G., D'aversa, F., Campanale, M. C., Cesario, V., Montalto, M., ... & Ojetti, V. (2013). Lactose intolerance: from diagnosis to correct management. European Review for Medical & Pharmacological Sciences, 17.
22. Shaw, A. D., & Davies, G. J. (1999). Lactose intolerance: problems in diagnosis and treatment. Journal of clinical gastroenterology, 28(3), 208-216.
23. Arola, H. (1994). Diagnosis of hypolactasia and lactose malabsorption. Scandinavian Journal of Gastroenterology, 29(sup202), 26-35.
24. Catanzaro, R., Sciuto, M., & Marotta, F. (2021). Lactose intolerance: An update on its pathogenesis, diagnosis, and treatment. Nutrition Research, 89, 23-34

25. Roxas, M. (2008). The role of enzyme supplementation in digestive disorders. Alternative medicine review, 13(4).
26. Wilt, T. J., Shaukat, A., Shamliyan, T., Taylor, B. C., MacDonald, R., Tacklind, J., ... & Levitt, M. (2010). Lactose intolerance and health. Evidence report/technology assessment, (192), 1-410.
27. Suarez, F. L., Savaiano, D. A., & Levitt, M. D. (1995). Review article the treatment of lactose intolerance. Alimentary pharmacology & therapeutics, 9(6), 589-597.
28. Montalto, M., Curigliano, V., Santoro, L., Vastola, M., Cammarota, G., Manna, R., ... & Gasbarrini, G. (2006). Management and treatment of lactose malabsorption. World journal of gastroenterology: WJG, 12(2), 187.
29. Szilagyi, A., & Ishayek, N. (2018). Lactose intolerance, dairy avoidance, and treatment options. Nutrients, 10(12), 1994.
30. Suarez, F. L., Savaiano, D. A., & Levitt, M. D. (1995). Review article the treatment of lactose intolerance. Alimentary pharmacology & therapeutics, 9(6), 589-597.
31. Petagna, L., Antonelli, A., Ganini, C., Bellato, V., Campanelli, M., Divizia, A., ... & Sica, G. S. (2020). Pathophysiology of Crohn's disease inflammation and recurrence. Biology direct, 15(1), 1-10.
32. Shanahan, F. (2001). Inflammatory bowel disease: immunodiagnostics, immunotherapeutics, and ecotherapeutics. Gastroenterology, 120(3), 622-635.
33. Shanahan, F. (2002). Crohn's disease. The Lancet, 359(9300), 62-69.

34. L, Neurath MF, Neumann H. Differential diagnosis in inflammatory bowel disease colitis: state of the art and future perspectives. World J Gastroenterol. 2015 Jan 7;21(1):21-46. doi: 10.3748/wjg.v21.i1.21. PMID: 25574078; PMCID: PMC4284336.
35. Sewell, G. W., Marks, D. J., & Segal, A. W. (2009). The immunopathogenesis of Crohn's disease: a three-stage model. Current opinion in immunology, 21(5), 506–513. https://doi.org/10.1016/j.coi.2009.06.003
36. Edwards, C. M., George, B. D., Jewell, D. P., Warren, B. F., Mortensen, N. J., & Kettlewell, M. G. (2000). Role of a defunctioning stoma in the management of large bowel Crohn's disease. The British journal of surgery, 87(8), 1063–1066. https://doi.org/10.1046/j.1365-2168.2000.01467.x
37. D'Haens GR, Geboes K, Peeters M, Baert F, Penninckx F, Rutgeerts P. Early lesions of recurrent Crohn's disease caused by infusion of intestinal contents in excluded ileum. Gastroenterology. 1998;114:262–267.
38. Gajendran, M., Loganathan, P., Jimenez, G., Catinella, A. P., Ng, N., Umapathy, C., ... & Hashash, J. G. (2019). A comprehensive review and update on ulcerative colitis. Disease-a-month, 65(12), 100851.
39. Langan, R. C., Gotsch, P. B., Krafczyk, M. A., & Skillinge, D. D. (2007). Ulcerative colitis: diagnosis and treatment. American family physician, 76(9), 1323-1330.
40. DeRoche, T. C., Xiao, S. Y., & Liu, X. (2014). Histological evaluation in ulcerative colitis. Gastroenterology report, 2(3), 178-192.

41. Farmer, R. G., Hawk, W. A., & Turnbull Jr, R. B. (1976). Indications for surgery in Crohn's disease: analysis of 500 cases. Gastroenterology, 71(2), 245-250.
42. Janowitz H. D. (1975). Problems in Crohn's disease: evaluation of the results of surgical treatments. Journal of chronic diseases, 28(2), 63–66. https://doi.org/10.1016/0021-9681(75)90062-4
43. Meier, J., & Sturm, A. (2011). Current treatment of ulcerative colitis. World journal of gastroenterology: WJG, 17(27), 3204.
44. Both, H., Torp-Pedersen, K., Kreiner, S., Hendriksen, C., & Binder, V. (1983). Clinical appearance at diagnosis of ulcerative colitis and Crohn's disease in a regional patient group. Scandinavian journal of gastroenterology, 18(7), 987–991. https://doi.org/10.3109/00365528309182127

9.

Inflammatory Bowel Disease and Mental Health

Dr Vijaita Gaur

Principal

SBN College of Education, Shri Madhopur

Email: gaurvijaita12@gmail.com

Abstract

Inflammatory bowel disease (IBD) is a chronic disorder of digestive tract. Ulcerative colitis, Crohn's disease and Micrscopic colitis are the major type of IBD disease. Diarrhea, fatigue, abdominal pain and cramping blood in stool etc symptoms occur in IBD disease. The physical health of IBD patients is affected by the symptoms and nature of the disease. This also affects the mental health of the patient. As a result of mental health disorders like stress, anxiety and depression arise. Psychotherapies like CBT, ACT, mindfulness based therapy etc. are used to treat these disorders.

Keywords: Disorder, Stress, Anxiety, Depression, Psychotherapies

1. Introduction

Inflammatory Bowel disease is basically related to digestive system and due to this disease many problem occur in human body. In this disease chronic inflammation occurs in gastrointestinal (GI) tract. There are most common two types, first Ulcerative colitis and second Crohn's disease. In Crohn's disease mouth to anus area affected of digestive tract means inflammation occurs in any part GI system and in ulcerative disease only colon and rectum area affected. Beside these types indeterminate colitis is the third type of inflammatory bowel disease. It has features of both type ulcerative colitis and crohn's disease.

2. Symptoms of IBD

IBD originate in the colon and rectum due to many reasons. This can affect other parts of the body and lead to IBD symptoms. The initial symptoms of IBD are caused by exposure to something that causes intestinal irritation such as a medication (including aspirin, ibuprofen and antibiotics) or GI infection. These symptoms go away but their effects on the immune system remain. Some common IBD symptoms given below-

Diarrhoea (sometime with blood)

Abdominal pain

Urgent need to defecate and incontinence

Rectal bleeding

Fever

Weigh loss

Anaemia

People who develop IBD in childhood have malnutrition and developmental delays.

3. Treatment of IBD

Treatment of inflammatory bowel disease focuses on reducing inflammation that triggers the patient's sign and symptoms. Most patient get relief from the symptoms of the disease but the risk of long term problem can also be reduced.IBD treatment involves drug therapy or surgery.

4. IBD and mental health

IBD impacts the quality of life patient. IBD can have a detrimental impact on patient lives due to the variety of severe symptomatology ranging from frequent bloody diarrhoea, accompanied by urgency to defecate and fecal incontinence, fatigue, abdominal pain and weight loss, to the early onset of the disease (15 to 30 year of age) disease fluctuation and lack of treatment. IBD is considered to negative effect due to which the daily routine of patient gets affected. Frequent illness leads to leave and unemployment. Along with the physical health of an IBD patient, the disease has significant impact on his mental health. The disease causes feeling of shame, isolation and physical dissatisfaction. As a result of these experiences, IBD patients are more likely to develop, stress, depression and anxiety, along with deterioration in the patient's physical health.

The relationship between IBD and mental health is not new. Historically, as early as the 1930s, gastroenterologists and psychiatrists recognized that events and experiences in a person's emotional life had a correlation between IBD disease and its severity. Therefore, at that time IBD was considered a psychosomatic disease and researchers conducted research studies related to it without considering the need for a control group in their studies. After a few decades, due to the lack of published studies and methodology in this area, it was considered a biological disease for some time, but research studies have indicated adverse effects of stressful experiences on IBD.

According Byrne et al. (2017) of anxiety and depression in IBD patients can be as high as 21% and 26% patient respectively. In another Cawthrope et al.(2015)found in their study that 82 % of people with ulcerative colitis and 54% of the general population were also diagnosed with mental disorder and in woman these disorders were more likely to occurs before or after ulcerative colitis ,but it is not necessary that every ulcerative colitis patient faces mental health.

Nahon et al. (2012) studied that actors like severe disease, low income source, not taking treatment as prescribed related to anxiety and factors like old age, active flares, physical disable, unemployed and low SES was also associated with depression in ulcerative colitis disorder. Qualter et al. (2020) studied the mental health of adolescents and young adult aged 14 to 25 with IBD.The result found that more severe disease was associated with poorer mental health. Additionally feeling of shame increase the risk of depression anxiety and loneliness in patient with IBD.Choi (2019) also found that the risk anxiety and depression increase after a diagnosis of IBD.

These findings show that IBD patients have relation with stress, anxiety depression and another mental health disorders. Patients also have an increased risk of anxiety, stress, and depression after diagnosis, indicating that the disease may contribute to anxiety and depression in many people

5. Symptoms of mental disorder

IBD is chronic bowel diseasc of GI System. There are mainly two types of Crohn's disease and ulcerative colitis. Medical conditions and causes of IBD disease. The mental health of the patient is also affected. In which stress, depression and anxiety mainly affect the patient. The following symptoms of stress, depression and anxiety appear in IBD patients.

5.1. Stress

Stress is a disorder arising from mental state. Stress arises due to imbalance and disharmony between mental state and situation. Stress is a conflict which creates a deep rift in the mind and emotions. Stress is gateway to many other mental disorders because in this the mind becomes disturbed, emotion become unstable and body feel unwell. In such a situation our efficiency get affected and our physical and mental development journey gets disrupted. IBD is a chronic disease that is challenging for the patient, including anxiety and stress about the disease and treatment. This disease will affect his family, relationships and work. There is pressure in his mind as to how he will be able to complete the tasks related to the above areas. Apart from this, irritability, depression or nervousness also occurs in the patient. Due to stress, the patient gets headache, fatigue and muscle aches etc symptoms like stress/pain also arise. Apart from this, feelings of anxiety, irritability, sadness and anger also arise.

5.2. Depression

In the field of psychology, depression is related to sadness related to emotions due to which it is considered a serious mood disorder in psychology. In this disease state, feelings of sadness arise along with loss of interest and one feels helpless, tired, feels helpless and disappointed.IBD disease which is a long term condition. In which this disease occurs during the pre- and post-treatment phase of the disease. The patient constantly looks sad and worried. His interest begins to wane and he does not find pleasure in activities related to these. He finds it difficult to concentrate, remember, take decisions as well as complete his tasks. Along with this, physical problems such as insomnia or excessive sleeping, low or high appetite and weight loss or weight gain. Problems like etc. restlessness, irritability and despair arise in the patient. As a result of these physical, mental and emotional changes, they develop feelings of negativity, feelings of guilt, worthlessness and helplessness. If person experience five or more of these symptoms for more than two weeks, encourage the person to seek evaluation from a professional clinical psychological counsellor.

5.3. Anxiety

Anxiety is a mental illness related to mental health in which a person worries excessively. Due to which he feels restlessness, fear or fear of something bad or bad happening, even though they have no real basis. In anxiety if a person suddenly becomes very nervous, he called panic attack. When obsessive compulsive disorders occur, it is called OCD and the stress disorder after trauma is called post-traumatic stress disorder. Anxiety has been observed in the pre- and post-treatment stages of IBD .The patient exhibits symptoms such as excessive worry, nervousness or feeling on edge and the person is not able to stop or control his or her anxiety. He worries too much about various things which affect his daily, professional and social life due to which he becomes restless and is afraid of bad things happening. These things make difficult to sit quietly and relax and do their work. He gets angry or irritable easily. If person experience five or more of these symptoms for more than two weeks, encourage the person to seek evaluation from a professional clinical psychological counsellor.

6. Curative Treatment of IBD Patients

When any psychological service is provided to a person or a client by a trained professional psychiatrist. This primarily uses forms of communication and interaction to assess, diagnose and treat emotional reactions, thinking patterns and behaviour patterns. This therapy is very useful for the treatment of behavioural problems of individuals. Various techniques are used in this therapy, such as experimental relationship-building, dialogue, communication and behaviour change etc. The psychotherapy may be provided to individuals, couples, families or members of a group. In this, during the therapy session, the trained professional tries to know about the patient's condition, mood, emotions, thoughts, behaviour and diagnose the problems and move the therapy forward.IBD patient have many behavioural problems like stress, depression and anxiety etc.These psychotherapies play important role in solving these problems in IBD patient and help to improve the quality of life and mental health which reflect physical health of IBD patient. So following psychotherapies used for IBD patient.

6.1. Cognitive behavioural therapy

In this therapy emphasis has been laid on the role of cognitive processes in the treatment of mental disorders like depression and anxiety, personality disorders, eating habits etc. This therapy was developed by Aaron Beck in the mid-1950s. This is an action-oriented approach. This therapy posits that the causes of many mental disorders may be directly related to cognitive problems. Beck believed that individuals are the product of the interaction of innate, biological, developmental, and environmental factors and those they have the capacity for self-determination. He believed that in mental disorders, the person misinterprets his signals and due to this misinterpretation, wrong thought patterns develop, which have a negative impact on the cognition and behaviour of the person. In this therapy, these undesirable thought patterns are identified and replaced with desirable thought patterns. In this, initially the therapist tries to promote positive relationships with the client. First of all the psychiatrist establishes a mutual relationship with the client, then he tries to help the person or patient identify his problem and after identifying the problem, a list of possible solutions is prepared by the patient. He then evaluates the positive and negative aspects of each solution. After that, he chooses the best solution from this list for implementation. In the therapeutic process, the client is encouraged to solve the problem. The therapist acts as a guide for the client by helping him understand his role in this. In this, the therapist not only tells the client that a particular belief is irrational, but by finding out the meaning, use and consequences associated with that irrational belief, these undesirable beliefs and thoughts are identified and challenged and they are transformed into objective, realistic and desirable ones. Thus, CBT improves the patient's quality of life by identifying the undesirable thought patterns and behaviours that cause depression and anxiety in IBD patients and converting them into desirable, positive behavioural thoughts.

6.2. Mindfulness based therapy

Mindfulness therapy is a type of talk psychotherapy. It consists of a conversation-based intervention. Through which the therapist makes a diagnosis by assessing the patient's dysfunctional thought patterns and behaviour and then provides treatment. In this, the client accepts everyday stressors, negative experiences and behaviours rather than ignoring them, and develops more desirable positive experiences and behaviours through the development of awareness by focusing on the present moment. There are also different types of mindfulness therapy, including mindfulness-based cognitive therapy (MBCT), mindfulness-based cognitive behavioural therapy (CBT), and mindfulness-based stress reduction therapy (MBSR). Additionally, mindfulness can also be incorporated into other forms of therapy. Mindfulness therapy uses many techniques such as meditation, body scan, breathing mindfulness stretching, yoga, sitting meditation, lengthen your exhale accept yourself, cultivating awareness, journaling etc.

6.3. Acceptance commitment therapy

This therapy was developed in 1999 by Steven Hayes. This is combination of behavioural Therapy and mindfulness based therapy (Behavioural Therapy + Mindfulness = ACT therapy). Its goal is to develop healthy and constructive activities committed to a positive attitude by accepting or consciously accepting cognitive distortions, negative unpleasant experiences and behaviours that are beyond one's control, without evaluating them or trying to change person do his or her work. It is very effective in anxiety and depression disorders. It contains 6 ACT processes (Cognitive defusion, Acceptance, Contact, the observing self, Value clarification, Commited action) by including which the client gets psychological flexibility. Due to these he can freely choose his actions keeping in mind his values despite his negative difficult thoughts and feelings. So along these lines ACT therapy was developed according this suggestion with the goal of teaching people that psychological pain is normal, and that we can learn ways to cope.

6.4. Gut-directed hypnotherapy

This therapy is a special form of hypnosis. This is based on the relationship between the mind and gut of the person. In this, therapy is done using suggestion, imagination and relaxation. A mind-body technique that aims to calm brain-gut communication by reducing unnecessary focus on body discomfort. Hypnotherapy uses tools that involve a trained professional bringing a person into a state of deep, relaxed concentration. It helps people by using their subconscious mind to change the way they think and act. This therapy helps IBD patients manage and live with IBD while overcoming their challenges and improving their quality of life with optimizes capacity.

6.5. Biofeedback

It is an alternative medical approach. It is also a mind body therapy that can improve a person's physical and mental health. In this, during the therapy session, the therapist uses non-invasive monitoring devices to measure the involuntary body movements of the client, like heart rate, breathing, sweat gland activity, skin temperature, pulse rate and muscle tension, etc. based on the feedback received from these devices, the therapist suggests to the patient how to by education and practice It also can have physical and medical benefits such as lowering blood pressure and improving pain control.

6.6. Stress reduction techniques

This process provides relaxation to a person by reducing the impact of stress on his mind and body. Stress and anxiety have a negative impact on IBD patients. These techniques help in dealing with stress and anxiety related to health problems like pain.

So these therapies are very useful for IBD patient. The relationship between mental health and psychotherapy techniques of IBD patients has been studied by researchers in many research works. Evertsz et al., (2017) studied that CBT is effective psychotherapy in improving QOL of IBD patient and also effective reducing anxiety and depression in IBD patient. Schoultz et al.,(2015)also studied that Mindfulness-based cognitive therapy has the potential to reduce depression and anxiety while improving the overall symptom management and quality of life of IBD patients. In 2011 INSPIRE study shows Stress management psychotherapy may not improve or reduce disease-related physical symptoms in IBD patients, but it may improve quality of life, especially in UC patients. Peerani et al., (2022) in a study of a 12-week online stress prevention intervention program, they found that the intervention had ameliorative effects on patient stress, mental health, and HRQoL but had no effect on IBD symptom indices. In 2002 Palsson et al.and in 2005 Tan and Hammond both found that Gut-directed hypnotherapy is well-tolerated and effective in irritable bowel syndrome. Brona, et al.(2019) found in a randomized controlled trial of patients with IBD, an 8-week ACT therapy course improved stress and other indices of psychological health.

7. Corrective measure to improve mental health

IBD is a disease of chronic nature. Sometime patient feels uncertain about the improvement in his disease when there is no reduction in the symptoms of his disease like digestive pain, diarrhoea etc. He thinks that he will not get relief from these symptoms and he feels isolated and alone. There are many changes occurs in the patient's body, lifestyle, activities etc in IBD disease. These changes arise some problems like pain, fatigue and many emotional problems in the patient. These are very difficult to express. This negatively impacts his physical health as well as his mental health. Therefore, the patient should take care of his mental health along with his physical health.IBD patients can also adopt the corrective measures given below for their mental health, which will have a positive impact on their mental as well as physical health .

1. Create or join peer groups or support groups so that person does not feel lonely.
2. Talk openly with your partner or loved ones and express your feelings, experiences and needs openly
3. For person mental problems, take the help of a trained professional psychiatrist who is familiar with the problems arising along with person physical problem and can help the patient in solving the mental problems arising due to it.
4. Learn management strategies from a psychiatrist to reduce anxiety, stress and depression.
5. Practice meditations in daily life.
6. Regular exercise has a great impact on mental health because exercise releases endorphin which improves a person's mood and reduces problems like depression, stress and anxiety.
7. Also do yoga regularly.
8. Give place to your interests like gardening, listening to songs etc. in your regular routine.
9. Follow your regular routine and get a regular sleep. Do not consume substances like caffeine etc. that interfere with sleep.
10. Eat a balanced diet as per the advice of a dietician.
11. Keep time for rest in your regular routine.
12. Use the medium of technical communication like phone call, video chat or social media in balanced quantity
13. Participate in social or workplace related programs and activities.
14. Do not be afraid of your workplace related or other programs and keep an emergency kit with you. Keep all the necessary items in it.

15. Express your thoughts through a diary or other means
16. Take care of yourself, focus on the present moment and do your work happily.
17. Keep a positive attitude.

References

1. Andrew, M., McCombie, Roger, T.,Mulder, Richard B., Gearry.(2013) Psychotherapy for inflammatory bowel disease: A review and update. *Journal of Crohn's and Colitis*, Volume 7, Issue 12, Pages 935–949
2. Barberio, B., Zamani ,M., Black, C.J., Savarino, E. V., Ford, A.C., (2021) Prevalence of symptoms of anxiety and depression in patients with inflammatory bowel disease: a systematic review and meta-analysis. *Lancet Gastroenterol Hepatol.* 6:359–70
3. Bennebroek, Evertsz F., Sprangers, MAG., Sitnikova, K., Stokkers, PCF., Ponsioen, CY. Bartelsman, JFWM., Van Bodegraven A.A., Fischer, S, Depla, ACTM., Mallant,RC, Sanderman, R., Burger, H., Bockting, CLH., (2017) Effectiveness of cognitive-behavioural therapy on quality of life, anxiety and depressive symptoms among patients with inflammatory bowel disease: A multicenter randomized controlled trial. *J Consult Clin Psychol*,85(9):918-925
4. Bernstein, CN., Zhang, L., Lix, LM., Graff, LA., Walker, JR., Fisk, JD., et al. (2018) The validity and reliability of screening measures for depression and

anxiety disorders in inflammatory bowel disease. *Inflammatory Bowel Dis.* 24:1867–75.

5. Boye, B., Lundin, KE., Jantschek, G., Leganger, S.,Mokleby, K., Tangen, T.,Jantschek, I,.Pripp, AH., Wojniusz, S., Dahlstroem, A., Rivenes, AC., Benninghoven, D., Hausken, T. Roseth, A., Kunzendorf, S., Wilhelmsen, I., Sharpe, M., Blomhoff, S., Malt, UF,.Jahnsen ,J., (2011)INSPIRE study: does stress management improve the course of inflammatory bowel disease and disease-specific quality of life in distressed patients with ulcerative colitis or Crohn's disease? A randomized controlled trial. *Inflammation Bowel Dis*, 17(9),1863-73.
6. Byrne, G., Rosenfeld, G., Leung, Y., et al.(2017) Prevalence of anxiety and depression in patients with inflammatory bowel disease.Can *J Gastroenterol Hepatol*,1–6.
7. Choi, K., Chun, J., Han, K., et al.(2019) Risk of anxiety and depression in patients with inflammatory bowel disease: a nationwide, population-based study. *J Clin Med.* 8(5),654.
8. Cawthorpe, David & Marta, Davidsom, MD., (2015) Temporal Co morbidity of Mental Disorder and Ulcerative. *The Permanente Journal*, 19(1);52-57
9. Emma, Paulides, Inge, Boukema., Christien, Janneke, V.W..Nanne, K.H.,Debore.,(2021) The Effect of Psychotherapy on Quality of life in IBD Patients: A Systematic Review. *Inflamm Bowel Disease*.Volume27,Issue5,Page711-724
10. Fulton, P., Germer, C., Siegel, R., (2005). Mindfulness and Psychotherapy; New York: Guilford Press.

11. Goodhand, JR., Wahed, M., Mawdsley, JE., Farmer, AD., Aziz, Q., Rampton, DS., (2012). Mood disorders in inflammatory bowel disease: Relation to diagnosis, disease activity, perceived stress, and other factors. Inflammatory Bowel Dis. 18:2301–9.
12. Jones, JL., Nguyen, GC., Benchimol, EI., et al. (2019) The impact of inflammatory bowel disease in Canada 2018: quality of life. *J Can Assoc Gastroenterol*.2:S42–S48.
13. Keefer, L., Taft, TH., Kiebles, JL., et al. (2013) Gut-directed hypnotherapy significantly augments clinical remission in quiescent ulcerative colitis. *Aliment Pharmacol Ther*. 761–71.
14. Klag, T., Mazurak, N., Fantasia, L.,et., (2017) High demand for psychotherapy in patient with inflammatory bowel disease. *Inflamm bowel disease*,1796-1802
15. Knowles, S.R., Keefer, L., Wilding, H., et al. (2018) Quality of life in inflammatory bowel disease: a systematic review and meta-analyses-part II. *Inflamm Bowel Dis*.966–976
16. Kochar, B. Barnes, EL. Long, MD. Cushing, KC. Galanko, J. Martin, CF. et al.(2018) Depression Is associated with more aggressive inflammatory bowel disease. *Am J Gastroenterol*. 113:80–5.
17. Krishnan,V.Nestler,EJ.(2008) The molecular neurobiology of depression. *Nature*, 455,894–902.
18. Kurina, LM., Goldacre, MJ., Yeates, D., Gill, LE.,(2001) Depression and anxiety in people with inflammatory bowel disease. *J Epidemiol Community Health*, 55,716–20.

19. Kutschera, M., Waldhor, T., Grochening, H.P., et al.(2000) The need for Psychological and Psychotherapeutic Intervention in Austrian patients with Inflammatory Bowl disease.
20. *J.Crohn Colitis*, 14:S308-309.
21. Leone, D. Gilardi, D.Corrò, BE. et al.(2019) Psychological characteristics of inflammatory bowel disease patients: a comparison between active and nonactive patients. *Inflamm Bowel Dis*,25:1399–1407.
22. Lesley, A., Graff, Rose, Geist., M., Ellen, Kuenzig., Eric, I., Benchimol, Gilaad, G., Kaplan, Joseph, W., Windsor, Alain., Bitton, Stephanie., Coward, Jennifer, L., Jones, Kate., Lee, Sanjay, K., Murthy, Juan-Nicolás,Peña-Sánchez, Laura, E., Targownik, Nazanin, Jannati, Tyrel., Jones, May., Tasbeen, Akhtar, Sheekha.Tal, Davis., Jake, Weinstein., Ghaida, Dahlwi., James, H. B., Im., Jessica, Amankwah, Osei. Noelle, Rohatinsky. Sara, Ghandeharian. Quinn, Goddard.Julia, Gorospe.Shira, Gertsman. Michelle,Louis., Richelle, Wagner., Colten, Brass., Rhonda, Sanderson., Charles, N. Bernstein.(2023) The 2023 Impact of Inflammatory Bowel Disease in Canada: Mental Health and Inflammatory Bowel Disease. *Journal of the Canadian Association of Gastroenterology,* Volume 6, Issue Supplement 2, Pages S64–S75,
23. Li, Z., Shang, W., Wang, C., Yang, K., Guo, J.(2022) Characteristics and trends in acceptance and commitment therapy research: A bibliometric analysis. *Front Psychol,* 14,13,980848.
24. Lores,T .,Goess, C., Mikocka-Walus, A., et al.(2020) Integrated psychological care reduces healthcare

costs at a hospital-based inflammatory bowel disease service. *Clin Gastroenterol Hepatol*, In press,

25. Lores,T.Goess, C., Mikocka-Walus, A., et al.(2019) Integrated psychological care is needed, welcomed and effective in ambulatory inflammatory bowel disease management: evaluation of a new initiative. *J Crohns Colitis*,13,819–827.
26. Mikocka-Walus, A., Andrews, JM.,(2018) It is high time to examine the psyche while treating IBD. *Nat Rev Gastroenterol Hepatol*, 15:329–30.
27. Mikocka-Walus, A., Pittet, V., Rossel, JB., Von, Känel R.,(2016) Symptoms of Depression and Anxiety Are Independently Associated With Clinical Recurrence of Inflammatory Bowel Disease. *Clin Gastroenterol Hepatol*, 14,829–35.
28. Nahon, S., Lahmek, P., Durance, C., Olympie, A., Lesgourgues, B.,Colombel, JF., et al..(2012) Risk factors of anxiety and depression in inflammatory bowel disease. *Inflamm Bowel Dis*, 18:2086–91.
29. Narula, N., Pinto-Sanchez, MI., Calo, N., Ford, AC., Bercik, P.,Reinisch, W., et al.(2019) Anxiety but not depression predicts poor outcomes in inflammatory bowel disease. *Inflamm Bowel Dis*, 25:1255–61.
30. Neale, JM., Davison, GC.,(2001) Abnormal psychology (8th ed.);New York: John Wiley & *Sons*, 247.
31. Neuendorf, R., Harding, A., Stello, N., Hanes, D.,Wahbeh, H., (2016) Depression and anxiety in patients with Inflammatory Bowel Disease: A systematic review. *J Psychosom Res*, 87:70–80.
32. Palsson, OS., Turner, MJ.,Johnson, DA., Burnett, CK., Whitehead,WE.,(2002) Hypnosis treatment for

severe irritable bowel syndrome: investigation of mechanism and effects on symptoms. *Digestive diseases and sciences.* 47,2605–14

33. Pamela, Qualter,.Alison, Rouncefield., Swales., Lucy, Bray.,Lucy, Blake.,Steven, Allen.Chris, Probert., Kay, Crook., & Bernie, Carter.,(2020)Depression ,anxiety and loneliness among adolescents and Young adults with in the UK; the role of disease severity, age of onset and embarrassment of the condition. *Quality of Life research*, Volume 30, page 497-506
34. Peerani, F., Watt, M., Ismond, KP., Whitlock, R., Ambrosio, L., Hotte, N., Mitchell, N., Bailey, RJ., Kroeker, K., Dieleman, LA., Siffledeen, J., Lim, A., Wong, K., Halloran, BP., Baumgart, DC., Taylor, L., Raman, M., Madsen, KL., Tandon, P., (2022) A randomized controlled trial of a multicomponent online stress reduction intervention in inflammatory bowel disease. *Therap Adv Gastroenterol*, 27,15:: 10..
35. Rachman, S., In, Clark. D., Fairburn, CG., Gelder, MG (eds.).,(1997) The evolution of cognitive behaviour therapy Science and practice of cognitive behaviour therapy. Oxford: *Oxford University Press*, pp. 1–26.
36. Riehl, E. Megan,(2018) The Emerging Role of Brain-Gut Therapies for Irritable Bowel Syndrome. *Gastroenterol Hepatol (N Y)*, 14(7): 436–438
37. Schoultz, M., Atherton, I., Watson, A.,(2015) Mindfulness-based cognitive therapy for inflammatory bowel disease patients: findings from an exploratory pilot randomised controlled trial. *Trials*, 25;16:379.
38. Sajadinejad, M., S. Asgari, K., Molavi, H., Kalantari ,M., Adibi, P.,(2012) Psychological Issues in

Inflammatory Bowel Disease: An Overview. *Gastroenterology Research and Practice*, vol,11 pages

39. Tan, G., Hammond, DC., Joseph, G., (2005) Hypnosis and irritable bowel syndrome: a review of efficacy and mechanism of action. *The American journal of clinical hypnosis. 47:161–78.*
40. Tiles-Sar, N., Neuser, J., De Sordi, D., Rücker, G., Baltes, A., Preiss, J., Moser, G., Timmer, A.,(2022) Psychological interventions for inflammatory bowel disease: a systematic review and component network meta-analysis protocol. *BMJ Open*, 22;12(6)
41. Trull, TJ., (2007). Clinical psychology; (7th ed.). Belmont, CA:
42. Van den Brink, G., Stapersma, L., Marroun, H. El., Henrichs,J., Szigethy, EM., Utens, EM., et al.(2016) Effectiveness of disease-specific cognitive-behavioural therapy on depression, anxiety, quality of life and the clinical course of disease in adolescents with inflammatory bowel disease: study protocol of a multicentre randomised controlled trial (HAPPY-IBD). *BMJ Open Gastroenterol,* 3:
43. Walker, JR., Ediger, JP., Graff, LA., Greenfeld, JM., Clara, I., Lix, L., et al.(2008) The Manitoba IBD cohort study: A population-based study of the prevalence of lifetime and 12-month anxiety and mood disorders. *Am J Gastroenterol,* 103:1989–97.
44. Worthen, M., Cash, E.,(2024) Stress Management. [Updated 2023 Aug 14]. In: StatPearls [Internet]. *Treasure Island (FL)*: StatPearls Publishing
45. Wynne,
Brona ., McHugh,Louise., Gao,Wei, Keegan.,Denise.,

Byrne, Kathryn .,Rowan, Catherine.,Hartery ,Karen., Kirschbaum,Clemens ., Doherty, Glen., Cullen, Garret., Dooley, Barbara., Mulcahy, Hugh. E., (2019) Acceptance and Commitment Therapy Reduces Psychological Stress in Patients With Inflammatory Bowel Diseases. *Gastroenterology*,Volume 156, Issue 4, Pages 935-945.e1

46. Yanartas, O., Kani, HT., Bicakci, E., Kilic, I., Banzragch, M., Acikel, C., et al.(2016) The effects of psychiatric treatment on depression, anxiety, quality of life, and sexual dysfunction in patients with inflammatory bowel disease. *Neuropsychiatrc Dis Treat*, 12:673–83.

List of Published Books

1. Gupta K and Jain M. Vridhopayogi Vyanjan: Vridhjano ke liye Upcharatmak Pak Vidhiyan. Abhinav Prakashan. Ajmer. 2016. ISBN: 978-938418946-4

This book contains more than 65 healthy food recipes developed, prepared and clinically verified by myself alone, tailored with the nutritional needs of the geriatric population.

2. Gupta K. Community Science and Sustainable Community Development. Lambart Academic Publication. Germany 2021. ISBN: 978-620419757-9

This book provides excellent research data related to different aspects of community which will be helpful to strengthen the sustainability of a community in terms of health, nutrition, wellness and economy.

3. Gupta K. 75 years of Indian Independence: Food and Nutritional Achievements, Opportunities and Challenges (Volume 1). Notion Press. Chennai. 2022. ISBN: 979-888883053-6

4. Gupta K. 75 years of Indian Independence: Food and Nutritional Achievements, Opportunities and Challenges (Volume 2). Notion Press. Chennai. 2022. ISBN: 979-888883757-3

5. Gupta K. 75 years of Indian Independence: Food and Nutritional Achievements, Opportunities and Challenges (Volume 3). Notion Press. Chennai. 2022. ISBN: 979-888909005-2

These three books provide enriched research data pertaining to various aspects of health, lifestyle, tourism, agriculture, antenatal or post natal diet, nutritional status, cognition and nutrition, etc., that will be extremely helpful to improve quality of life of the individuals ultimately making healthy and sustainable community.

6. Gupta K. Aazadi ka Amrit Mahotsav: Community Science Achievements, Opportunities and Challenges. BlueRose One Publishers. India. 2023. ISBN: 978-935704938-2

This book is particularly based on different disciplines of community science, i.e., food science and nutrition, food security, advancement in food preservation and processing, sustainable breeding and cultivation approaches in agriculture, importance of prebiotics, role of therapeutic diet, importance of nutrition for pregnant ladies and children, how cognitive development is affected by nutritional status of the children, spiritual development, skill based learning system DEASA, effect of social media on community development.

7. Gupta K. Nutrition Education: An Important Pillar of Health. Notion Press. Chennai. 2023. ISBN: 979-888959915-9

This book is particularly based on different topics of nutrition science, i.e., importance of nutrition in daily life, flavours of Bengal, flavours of Ramadan, Indian spices, celebrate a world of flavours, nutrition in bed bound patients, why nutrition is essential and importance of homemade pickles in daily diet.

8. Gupta K, Bhushan V, Pandey A. Issues with Girls. Notion Press. Chennai. 2023. ISBN: 979-889026221-9

This book is particularly based on different topics related to girls and women, i.e., change in education to bring empowerment, mental hygiene, health and diet management, rise in health problems: A wake up call, girls hygiene and nutrients, letting the girls grow naturally, nutrition for girls, optimal nutrition, good health and wellbeing,: are we there yet?, women's leadership and role model for girls, empowering girls: dare to dream, baby girl: beautiful miracles.

9. Gupta K, Tripathi KM, Meena N, Sukhwal I, Soni V. Recent Trends in Community Science. BlueRose One Publishers. India. 2023. ISBN: 978-935819026-7

This book is based on different area of community science, i.e., parenting techniques and changes in parenting over the time, association between eating out and childhood obesity, rural participation and community development, ergonomics for everyone, kitchen ergonomics, use of unconventional fibres in textile industry, sustainable techniques for dye application (textile industry), spiritual development, therapeutic nutrition, impact of dietary habits on people suffering from polycystic ovarian syndrome (PCOS), millets: heritage of India, *terminalia arjuna* herb and its impact on hypercholesterolemia's patients, black cumin seeds, development disorders of children and homoeopathic treatment, success stories of women entrepreneurs from fields of community science.

10. Gupta K, Katiyar P, Meena S, Tripathi KM,. Millets: The Miracle of Nature. Notion Press. Chennai. 2023. ISBN: 979-889066606-2

This book is particularly based on topics such as millets- the nutria-cereal, magical grains, millets- the climate resilient nutria cereals, India's treasury: millets as dietary accessory, therapeutic role of millets in daily life, nutritional impact of millets on pregnant mothers, economic aspects of millets etc,.

11. Gupta K, Cherian B, Ramalakshmi, Harjai K. Health and Wellness (A basic guide to obtain good health). Notion Press. Chennai. 2023. ISBN: 979-889067222-3

Chapters of this book entitled "Health and Wellness (A basic guide to obtain good health)" particularly based on topics such as Blood, breathing & thoughts, Meditation, yoga, silence and prayer, Mind-body connection: Using yoga to enhance maternal health, Improve your low self-esteem with blessings of yoga and meditation, Food habits, Nutrition for health, Biogreens: the immunity booster, Role of nutrition in obesity, No health without mental health, Ayurveda for holistic health care, Homoeopathic biochemic treatment, Palliative care, Functional foods in cardiovascular disease, Union government initiatives to provide affordable, accessible, and quality healthcare for all.

12. Gupta K, Gaur V, Kumari R, Mishra S, Arya L, Mukharjee G. Health for All. Notion Press. Chennai. 2023. ISBN: 979-889133024-5

The edited book volume is primarily intended to be a collection of peer reviewed and plagiarism free chapters written by research scholars, academicians, scientists, doctors and faculty members of their respective fields. Chapters of this book entitled "Health for All" particularly based on topics such as sustainable innovation strategies in public health, application of technology in healthcare, world health organization's policies on world nutrition, the invisible threat of food borne diseases, obesity in affluent societies and its effect, role of nutrition education, treatment of diseases using different medical systems, non communicable diseases through workplace wellness initiatives, immunization program and serum banking in India.

13. Gupta K, Swamy D, Jain S, Sangeeta, Rochani C, Verma R. Current Advances in Community Science. Notion Press. Chennai. 2023. ISBN: 979-889186087-2

The edited book volume is primarily intended to be a collection of peer reviewed and plagiarism free chapters particularly based on topics such as impact and benefits of nano-fertilizers, understanding the benefits of dietary fibres on health, importance of food fortification, consumer problems and protection in India related to adulteration, black marketing, health and psychological well-being, role of millets to sustain food and nutritional security, extension education in modern era, paradigm shift in extension approaches for sustainable development, computer aided designing in textiles and apparel industry, use of microfibers, Instagram as a tool to promote micro apparels and qualitative analysis on the different areas of skill development in community science.

14. Gupta K, Katiyar P, Verma P, Pawar RV, Sangeeta. Food Safety & Security- A Basic Guide. Notion Press. Chennai. 2023. ISBN: 979-889233007-7

Chapters of this book entitled "Food safety and food security (A basic guide)" particularly based on topics such as foodborne diseases, immunity boosters, feeding the nation, when food turns foul, national and international organizations working for food safety, food spoilage, food poisoning, food preservation, food safety, food security, food safety and standard authority of India (FSSAI), natural farming, food standards, food safety risk assessment and management, role of government in ensuring food safety, role of food pickles in achieving household food security, assessing the benefits and costs of improving food safety.

15. Gupta K, Venkatappa KG, Devi KV, Sangeeta, Pal P. Brain: Associations, Wellness & Treatment. Notion Press. Chennai. 2024. ISBN: 979-889233671-0

Chapters of this book entitled **"Brain: Associations, Wellness and Treatment"** particularly based on topics such as brain health and disabilities, what I learnt about our brain, heads off to migraine, effect of stress on mental health, unlocking mental wellness, Parkinson's disease and its homeopathic treatment, mental health, depression, interrelation between brain health and cognitive functioning, artificial intelligence and cognitive science, effect of sleep patterns on brain health, prioritizing brain health, spirituality and brain health, impact of financial condition on brain heath, drugs and brain health; and impact of homemade food on maintaining brain health and wellness.

16. Gupta K, Mukharjee G, Esaivani KB, Sangeeta, Anuradha K, Jethwani P. Handbook on Inflammatory Bowel Disease (Volume 1). Hemakshee Publication. Sikar. 2024 ISBN: 978-81-969920-0-2

This book titled **"Handbook on Inflammatory Bowel Disease (Volume 1)"** is primarily intended to be a collection of peer reviewed and plagiarism free chapters written by research scholars, academicians, scientists, doctors and faculty members of their respective fields. Chapters of this book particularly based on topics such as etiology differential diagnosis, prevention and treatment of inflammatory bowel disease (IBD); malnutrition and IBD, role of yoga & meditation in IBD, yoga techniques & quality of life in patients with IBD, role of diet in IBD, use of micro-organisms in prevention & treatment of IBD, role of remission diet in IBD and pediatric IBD compass.

17. Gupta K, Annapurna A, Verma P, Pal P, Supriya. Nurturing Bonds: A Holistic Guide to Breastfeeding Bliss. Hemakshee Publication. Sikar. 2024. ISBN: 978-81-969920-3-3.

Chapters of this book entitled **"Nurturing Bonds: A Holistic Guide to Breastfeeding Bliss"** particularly based on topics such as importance of breastfeeding to child and mothers, nurturing our future, infant food, promote breastfeeding, lactation and solemnization of the bond of motherhood, importance of breastfeeding- a holistic approach, nourishing empowerment, the significance of breastfeeding: a comprehensive comparison with infant formula feeding, breastfeeding in special circumstances, breastfeeding support in India, a mother's journey through breastfeeding, etc.

Note: These books are available on publisher's website, Amazon and FlipKart

www.ingramcontent.com/pod-product-compliance
Ingram Content Group UK Ltd.
Pitfield, Milton Keynes, MK11 3LW, UK
UKHW021402190726
13845UKWH00028B/832

9 788196 992019